International Cardio-Oncology Society (IC-OS) Board Review Manual

A Guide to Cardio-Oncology

Volume 2

AF837245

IC-OS
International
Cardio-Oncology
Society

International Cardio-Oncology Society

International Cardio-Oncology Society (IC-OS) Board Review Manual

A Guide to Cardio-Oncology

Volume 2

Editors

Jose A. Alvarez-Cardona, MD
Assistant Professor of Medicine
Leon H. Charney Division of Cardiology
New York University School of Medicine
NYU Langone Health
New York, New York, USA

Daniel J. Lenihan, MD
Immediate Past President and Founder,
International Cardio-Oncology Society
Saint Francis Healthcare
Cape Girardeau, Missouri, USA

Arjun K. Ghosh, MBBS, MSc, PhD
Consultant Cardiologist
Barts Heart Centre (BHC)
St. Bartholomew's Hospital
University College London Hospital (UCLH)
London, United Kingdom

IC-OS
International
Cardio-Oncology
Society

International Cardio-Oncology Society

ISBN: 978-1-7356442-2-6

Library of Congress Control Number:

Typeset by Brih Inc.

First Edition 2020

International Cardio-Oncology Society
602 Audubon Ave, Tampa, Florida 33609 USA

http://www.ic-os.org

Preface

It has become quite apparent that *Cardio-Oncology* has arrived and important developments in this discipline of medicine are occurring at an astonishing rate. It is clearly evident that all aspects of contemporary cancer therapeutics are rapidly progressing and the success of these therapies has been quite impressive to say the least. We are very excited to provide an up-to-date review for the state of *Cardio-Oncology*.

The IC-OS Board Review Manual: A Guide to *Cardio-Oncology* is a compilation of board-style questions and evidence-based explanations designed by experts from around the world to guide clinicians through the developing discipline of *Cardio-Oncology*. This book is part of a global effort to create awareness about the cardiovascular care of the patient with cancer and to promote new scientific endeavors. It is also intended to help healthcare providers prepare for the certification exam administered by the International Cardio-Oncology Society (IC-OS).

Jose A. Alvarez-Cardona, MD
Daniel J. Lenihan, MD
Arjun K. Ghosh, MBBS, MSc, PhD

Contributors

Ana Barac, MD PhD
D'Aniello Chair and Medical Director of Cardio-Oncology
Inovar Schar Cancer Center and Inova Heart and Vascular Institute
Fairfax, Virginia, USA

Andrés Daniele, MD
Chair, Department of Cardio-Oncology
Instituto de Oncología Ángel H. Roffo
Buenos Aires, Argentina

Anju Nohria, MD, MSc
Associate Professor of Medicine
Director, Cardio-Oncology Program
Dana-Farber Cancer Institute
Brigham and Women's Hospital/ Harvard Medical School
Boston, Massachusetts, USA

Anne Blaes, MD
Professor of Medicine
Director, Division of Hematology, Oncology, and Transplantation
Director of Cancer Survivorship Services and Translational Research
Masonic Cancer Center
University of Minnesota
Minneapolis, Minnesota, USA

Charles B. Porter, MD
Professor of Medicine
Director, Cardio-Oncology Program
University of Kansas Medical Center
Kansas City, Kansas, USA

Dipti Gupta, MD, MPH
Assistant Professor of Medicine
Program Director, Cardio-Oncology Clinical Research Fellowship
Memorial Sloan Kettering Cancer Center
Weill Cornell Medical College
New York, New York, USA

Iskra Pusic, MD
Associate Professor of Medicine
Oncology Division, Section of Bone Marrow Transplantation & Leukemia
Washington University School of Medicine
Saint Louis, Missouri, USA

Jennifer Liu, MD
Professor of Medicine
Chief, Cardiology Service at Memorial Sloan Kettering Cancer Center
Weill Cornell Medical College
New York, New York, USA

Joerg Herrmann, MD
Professor of Medicine
Director, Cardio-Oncology Program
Chair, Research Division of Ischemic Heart Disease and Critical Care
Consultant, Division of Cardiovascular Medicine
Mayo Clinic College of Medicine and Science
Rochester, Minnesota, USA

Joseph R. Carver, MD
Chief of Staff, Abramson Cancer Center
Emeritus Director, Thalheimer Center for Cardio-Oncology
Bernard Fishman Clinical Professor of Medicine
University of Pennsylvania School of Medicine
Philadelphia, Pennsylvania, USA

Michael Fradley, MD
Associate Professor of Medicine
Medical Director, Thalheimer Center for Cardio-Oncology
Section Chief, Consultative Cardiology
University of Pennsylvania School of Medicine
Pennsylvania, Philadelphia, USA

Richard K. Cheng, MD, MSc
Associate Professor of Medicine, Division of Cardiology
Adjunct Associate Professor of Radiology
University of Washington Medical Center
Seattle, Washington, USA

Sebastian Szmit, MD, PhD
President, International Cardio-Oncology Society Poland Chapter
Associate Professor of Medicine
Centre of Postgraduate Medical Education (CMKP)
Warsaw, Poland

Susan F. Dent, MD
Current President, International Cardio-Oncology Society
Professor of Medicine
Associate Director of Breast Cancer Clinical Research
Co-Director of Cardio-Oncology program
Duke University School of Medicine and Duke Health
Durham, North Carolina, USA

Teresa López Fernández, MD
Chairperson Elect, European Society of Cardiology Council of Cardio-Oncology
Director, Cardio-Oncology Program
La Paz University Hospital
Madrid, Spain

Vijay Rao, MD, PhD
Director, Cardio-Oncology
Director, Heart Failure
Co-Director, Anticoagulation Clinic
Franciscan St. Francis Health
Indianapolis, Indiana, USA

Abbreviations

ASCO	American Society of Clinical Oncology
BNP	brain natriuretic peptide
CAR T	chimeric antigen receptor T-cell
CXR	chest X-ray
CV	cardiovascular
ECG	electrocardiogram
ED	Emergency Department
ER	estrogen receptor
Gy	Gray
HER2	human epidermal growth factor receptor 2
hs-CRP	high-sensitivity C-reactive protein
IL-6	interleukin-6
LVEF	left ventricular ejection fraction
NT-proBNP	N-terminal pro-brain natriuretic peptide
PR	progesterone receptor
R-CHOP	rituximab, cyclophosphamide, doxorubicin, vincristine, prednisone
TnI	troponin I
TnT	troponin T

Table of Contents

Questions Only

1. A 45-year-old male with essential hypertension presents with fatigue and exertional dyspnea. He was diagnosed with nodular sclerosis Hodgkin lymphoma at the age of 16 years and achieved his first remission after 6 cycles of ABVD (Adriamycin [doxorubicin], 300 mg/m^2; bleomycin, 120 units/m^2; vinblastine, 72 mg/m^2; and dacarbazine, 4.5 g/m^2), followed by 4000 centigray (cGy) mediastinal radiation. The patient relapsed after 6 months, received ICE (ifosfamide, cyclophosphamide, and etoposide), and subsequently underwent autologous stem cell transplantation. He then achieved complete remission. Which of the following element(s) of the patient's history is/are associated with the greatest long-term risk of heart failure?

   A. Bleomycin, dacarbazine
   B. Doxorubicin, mediastinal radiation
   C. Gender, autologous stem cell transplantation
   D. Vinblastine, age 45 years

2. Cytokine release syndrome (CRS) can occur after chimeric antigen receptor-T cell (CAR-T) treatment. Which of the following is a correct statement?

   A. A significant decrease in LVEF (left ventricular ejection fraction) can occur with any grade of CRS.
   B. Pre-existing treatment with anthracyclines is a contraindication to CAR-T therapy.
   C. Troponin level does not correlate with the grade of CRS.
   D. When CRS occurs, the early use of tocilizumab is associated with a lower rate of cardiovascular events.

3. A 64-year-old male with history of Philadelphia chromosome positive acute lymphoblastic leukemia undergoes hematopoietic stem cell transplantation. His conditioning regimen included busulfan and cyclophosphamide. Post-transplant, he is started on dasatinib maintenance therapy. In addition, he is receiving immunosuppression with tacrolimus. He missed two appointments for his blood work. He now presents with shortness of breath, tremors, lower extremity edema, and acute kidney injury with creatinine of 2.5 mg/dL (previously 0.7 mg/dL). There are schistocytes on peripheral smear review and there is a new reduction in his platelet count. What drug is the most likely cause of his presentation?

   A. Busulfan
   B. Cyclophosphamide
   C. Dasatinib
   D. Tacrolimus

4. Which of the following cardiac abnormalities carries the highest risk in the Hematopoietic Cell Transplantation-Specific Comorbidity Index?

   A. Arrhythmia
   B. Congestive heart failure
   C. Coronary artery disease
   D. Valvular disease (except asymptomatic mitral valve prolapse)

5. Which of the following statements is most correct regarding Chimeric Antigen Receptor (CAR) T-cell therapy?

   A. Life-threatening hemodynamic instability and cardiogenic shock is usually attributed to Cytokine Release Syndrome (CRS) after CAR T-cell therapy.
   B. Multiple studies have shown that cardiovascular manifestations of CRS are due to off-target cross-reactivity of T-cell receptors against the striated muscle-specific protein.
   C. Routine monitoring of NT-proBNP or BNP level in patients receiving CAR T-cell therapy helps identify patients for early tocilizumab administration
   D. Steroids are routinely given to prevent the development of CRS after CAR T-cell therapy.

6. Which of the following statements is true regarding cardiac tumors?

   A. Cardiac rhabdomyosarcoma is the most common primary cardiac tumor in adults.
   B. Compared to metastatic cardiac tumors, primary cardiac tumors are more common.
   C. Primary malignant cardiac masses are most commonly found in the right atrium and pericardium.
   D. The majority of primary cardiac tumors are malignant.

7. Which of the following malignancies rarely metastasizes to the heart?

   A. Breast cancer
   B. Lung cancer
   C. Melanoma
   D. Prostate cancer

8. Which of the following syndromes is associated with cardiac myxomas?

   A. Carney complex
   B. Gorlin syndrome
   C. Li-Fraumeni syndrome
   D. Tuberous sclerosis

9. Which of the findings below, in the setting of high clinical suspicion for amyloid cardiomyopathy, is most specific for AL (light chain) amyloidosis?

   A. Interventricular septum measuring >1.2 centimeters (cm)
   B. Carpal tunnel syndrome

C. Macroglossia
D. Prominent cardiac uptake on pyrophosphate scan

10. Based on the Childhood Cancer Survivor Study (CCSS), childhood cancer survivors are at increased risk for heart failure, myocardial infarction, pericardial, and valvular disease. Which of the following factors has been shown to have a statistically significant association with all of these cardiovascular events?

    A. Doxorubicin therapy with a cumulative dose greater than 250 mg/m^2
    B. History of lymphoma
    C. Radiotherapy dose
    D. Younger age at diagnosis (before the age of 10 years)

11. A 29-year-old female presents with acute systolic heart failure and atrial fibrillation. Upon further questioning, the patient informed us that she was treated for lymphoma as a child. Which of the following may have contributed to the patient's current condition?

    A. Cisplatin
    B. Cyclophosphamide
    C. Dacarbazine
    D. Doxorubicin

12. Anthracycline use has been associated with significant cardiac dysfunction. Which of the following treatments has been shown to be effective at primary prevention of cardiac dysfunction?

    A. Carvedilol
    B. Dexrazoxane
    C. Enalapril
    D. Sacubitril-valsartan

13. A 26-year-old male with history of Hodgkin lymphoma at the age of 12 years was referred to the Cardio-Oncology Clinic for cardiovascular surveillance. He was treated with 4 courses of ABVE (doxorubicin [cumulative dose 200 mg/m^2], bleomycin, vincristine, and etoposide) in addition to mantle field radiation therapy. The patient is asymptomatic. He has stage 2 hypertension. A lipid panel demonstrates an elevated LDL 146 mg/dL (3.78 mmol/L). His body mass index is 28 kg/m^2 and has no family history of cardiovascular disease. Carotid Doppler ultrasound demonstrates mild atherosclerotic disease of the right external carotid artery. In addition to lifestyle modification, which of the following is the best treatment option for this patient?

    A. Observation and reassess his blood pressure and lipid panel in 3-6 months
    B. Start fish oil and pharmacologic antihypertensive therapy
    C. Start pharmacologic antihypertensive therapy and niacin
    D. Start pharmacologic antihypertensive therapy and statin therapy

14. A 69-year-old female with metastatic invasive ductal carcinoma of the right breast was referred to the Cardio-oncology clinic before starting trastuzumab. Five years ago, she received anthracycline-based therapy for triple negative (HER2 negative, estrogen receptor negative, and progesterone receptor negative) breast cancer. One year after anthracycline therapy she developed mild symptomatic heart failure with a left ventricular ejection fraction (LVEF) of 38% and was started on enalapril and carvedilol. A new transthoracic echocardiogram reveals a non-dilated left ventricle with LVEF of 49%. The patient is asymptomatic (NYHA class 1 symptoms). Which of the following statements is true regarding the use of trastuzumab in this patient?

    A. Invasive coronary angiography should be performed prior to initiating trastuzumab.
    B. She can start trastuzumab since she has a low risk of developing cardiac dysfunction.
    C. The patient can be started on trastuzumab with close cardiac safety morning.
    D. Trastuzumab is contraindicated.

15. A 56-year-old male with melanoma presents with palpitations and chest pain. He was started on pembrolizumab 4 weeks ago. Transthoracic echocardiogram showed a normal left ventricular ejection fraction. Cardiac troponin is mildly elevated. Electrocardiogram was unremarkable. What would be the best next diagnostic test?

    A. Cardiac magnetic resonance imaging (MRI)
    B. Dobutamine stress echocardiogram
    C. Endomyocardial biopsy
    D. Transesophageal echocardiogram

16. A 58-year-old female with history of hypertension and diabetes is currently receiving doxorubicin-containing chemotherapy for breast cancer. Her baseline echocardiogram shows a normal left ventricular ejection fraction (LVEF) of 63% and global longitudinal strain (GLS) of -21%. An echocardiogram was obtained after the patient presented with shortness of breath and it showed a decrease in LVEF to 56% and GLS to -15%. Select the correct statement regarding a reduction in GLS. Select the correct statement regarding the clinical significance of a reduction in GLS.

    A. A reduction in GLS during treatment has no clinical significance if the LVEF remains normal.
    B. A reduction in GLS from -21% to -15.0% is indicative of subclinical LV dysfunction.
    C. GLS decline >25% correlates with a reduction in LVEF at 1 year.
    D. Temporarily hold cancer treatment until GLS improves

17. Which of the following modalities is preferred if 2-dimensional transthoracic echocardiography provides inaccurate or discrepant measurements of left ventricular systolic function due to poor image quality?

A. Cardiac magnetic resonance imaging (MRI)
B. Contrast-enhanced gated cardiac computed tomography (CT)
C. Non-contrast 3-dimensional echocardiography
D. Nuclear multigated acquisition scan (MUGA)

18. For a patient receiving trastuzumab and being monitored by echocardiography every 3 months, which of the following scenarios is most suggestive of subclinical left ventricular dysfunction?

A. A relative decrease in GLS by 15% compared to baseline
B. A relative increase in GLS by 15% compared to baseline
C. An absolute decrease in global longitudinal strain (GLS) from -20% to -18%
D. An absolute increase in GLS from -18% to -23%

19. Which of the following statements is true regarding the presence coronary artery calcification in patients with cancer?

A. A high coronary artery calcium (CAC) score is associated with a lower risk of cardiovascular events in women with breast cancer.
B. Current guidelines recommend obtaining a CAC score 2 years after thoracic radiotherapy.
C. The main limitation of the CAC score is exposure to a high radiation dose.
D. The presence of CAC on a staging CT chest can be used to determine cardiovascular risk.

20. A 48-year-old female with metastatic non-small cell lung cancer (anaplastic lymphoma kinase [ALK] positive) diagnosed 6 months ago presents to clinic complaining of dizziness and fatigue. Her vital signs revealed a blood pressure 110/60 mmHg, pulse 35 beats per minute (bpm), respiratory rate 10 breaths per minute, afebrile, and oxygen saturation 98% on room air. A 12-lead electrocardiogram demonstrated sinus bradycardia with a heart rate of 33 bpm. Which of the following treatments could potentially explain the patient's current presentation?

A. Bevacizumab
B. Crizotinib
C. Lenvatinib
D. Osimertinib

21. A 55-year-old male with chronic lymphocytic leukemia (CLL) is started on ibrutinib. Which of the following best describes its mechanism of action?

A. BCR-ABL kinase inhibitor
B. Cyclin-dependent kinase (CDK) inhibitor of CDK4 and 6
C. JAK tyrosine kinase inhibitor
D. Small-molecule inhibitor of Bruton's tyrosine kinase

22. Which of the following is an anti-CD38 monoclonal antibody used to treat multiple myeloma?

    A. Bevacizumab
    B. Carfilzomib
    C. Daratumumab
    D. Rituximab

23. A 65-year-old male was diagnosed with metastatic prostate cancer and is started on abiraterone. His grandson, who is a medical student, would like to know the drug's mechanism of action and potential adverse effects. Which of the following best describes abiraterone's mechanism of action and cardiovascular adverse effect profile?

    A. A gonadotropin releasing hormone (GnRH) agonist – increased risk of myocardial infarction
    B. A gonadotropin releasing hormone (GnRH) antagonist – QT interval prolongation
    C. An androgen biosynthesis inhibitor – hypertension
    D. An androgen receptor inhibitor – metabolic syndrome

24. Which of the following cancer drugs is associated with arterial thrombosis?

    A. Arsenic trioxide
    B. Bleomycin
    C. Ifosfamide
    D. Pazopanib

25. An 83-year-old female with myelodysplastic syndrome who receives blood transfusions periodically presents with worsening dyspnea on exertion. Vital signs show a pulse of 105 beats per minute, blood pressure of 110/80 mmHg, respiratory rate 18 breaths per minute, and oxygen saturation 98% on 2 liters per minute of supplemental oxygen via nasal cannula. Physical exam demonstrates an elevated jugular venous pressure and bilateral fine crackles with decreased breath sounds. Her N-terminal pro-brain natriuretic peptide (NT-proBNP), ferritin, and transferrin saturation are elevated. Which of the following tests will be most helpful in establishing the etiology of her presentation?

    A. Cardiac magnetic resonance imaging (MRI)
    B. Echocardiogram with strain imaging
    C. FDG/PET scan
    D. Pyrophosphate scan

26. A 73-year-old female with history of sinus node dysfunction is diagnosed with invasive ductal carcinoma of the left breast. Adjuvant radiation therapy is recommended. She has a left-sided dual chamber pacemaker and her ventricular pacing burden is 60%. Which of the following is most associated with radiation-induced device malfunction?

A. Anatomical location of the tumor (below diaphragm versus above diaphragm)
B. Cumulative tumor dose
C. Fraction of radiation therapy courses
D. High beam energy (≥15 megavolt [MV])

27. Which of the following is the proposed mechanism for ibrutinib-induced atrial fibrillation?

A. Decreased resveratrol production
B. Enhanced potassium channel blockade
C. Inhibition of C-terminal SRC kinase
D. Inhibition of platelet-derived growth factor (PDGF) signaling

28. Which of the following is considered a clinically acceptable maximum radiation dose to pacemakers and defibrillators?

A. 2 to 5 grays (Gy)
B. 11 to 20 Gy
C. 25 to 30 Gy
D. Less than 1 Gy

29. Which of the following cancer types has the highest points when calculating the Khorana score?

A. Lung
B. Lymphoma
C. Pancreas
D. Prostate

30. Which of the following oral anticoagulants have been effective at primary prevention of venous thromboembolism in patients with cancer and a Khorana score of ≥2?

A. Apixaban and dabigatran
B. Apixaban and rivaroxaban
C. Edoxaban and dabigatran
D. Edoxaban and rivaroxaban

31. In which of the following cases is prophylaxis for venous thromboembolism recommended by the American Society of Clinical Oncology?

A. Breast cancer treatment with exemestane
B. Melanoma treatment with nivolumab and ipilimumab
C. Multiple myeloma treatment with lenalidomide
D. Non-small cell lung cancer treatment with bevacizumab

32. A 64-year-old male with angioimmunoblastic T-cell lymphoma presents with worsening shortness of breath. He was treated with CHOP (cyclophosphamide, doxorubicin, vincristine, and prednisone), and 2 months later with BEAM (carmustine, etoposide, cytarabine, and melphalan) conditioning and autologous stem cell transplantation. A transthoracic echocardiogram was unremarkable. A chest CT scan 3 weeks after the transplant showed bilateral upper lobe ground-glass opacities and scattered pulmonary nodules. Vital signs revealed a pulse of 95 beats per minute, blood pressure of 110/60 mmHg, afebrile, and oxygen saturation of 93% on room air. Which of the following could explain the patient's clinical presentation?

    A. Carmustine
    B. Cyclophosphamide
    C. Doxorubicin
    D. Vincristine

33. Compared with dalteparin (low molecular weight heparin), which of the following statements is true regarding the use of an oral factor Xa inhibitor (rivaroxaban) in patients with cancer with venous thromboembolism (VTE)?

    A. Rivaroxaban is associated with a higher 6-month cumulative rate of VTE recurrence and non-major bleeding.
    B. Rivaroxaban is associated with a higher 6-month cumulative rate of VTE recurrence, but a lower rate of non-major bleeding.
    C. Rivaroxaban is associated with a lower 6-month cumulative rate of VTE recurrence, but a higher rate of non-major bleeding.
    D. Rivaroxaban is associated with lower 6-month cumulative rate of VTE recurrence and non-major bleeding.

34. According to the American College of Cardiology and American Heart Association, in what stage of heart failure should asymptomatic patients with no structural heart disease receiving anticancer therapies known to be associated with cardiotoxicity should be classified?

    A. Stage A
    B. Stage B
    C. Stage C
    D. Stage D

35. Which of the following iron chelators may be useful to prevent cardiac dysfunction in patients receiving doxorubicin?

    A. Deferasirox
    B. Deferiprone
    C. Deferoxamine
    D. Dexrazoxane

36. Compared to photon therapy, which of the following is true regarding the use of proton therapy in patients with cancer?

A. Proton therapy has been shown to improve overall survival in patients with locally advanced cancer.
B. Proton therapy is associated with a reduction in adverse effects.
C. Proton therapy results in a higher risk of decline in performance status.
D. Proton therapy results in a similar amount of radiation exposure.

37. Which of the following statements is correct regarding radiation-induced heart disease?

A. Right-sided cardiac valves are more often involved versus left-sided.
B. The extent of aorto-mitral curtain thickening and/or calcification is associated with surgical mortality.
C. The left bundle branch is more susceptible to the effects of radiation than the right bundle branch.
D. Valvular heart disease usually manifests earlier than coronary artery disease.

38. Which of the following genetic mutations associated with the development of a dilated cardiomyopathy has also been found to carry a higher risk for the development of anthracycline-induced cardiotoxicity?

A. Lamin A/C (LMNA)
B. Sodium channel SCN5A
C. Titin-truncating variants
D. TNNT2

39. Which of the following statements is most accurate regarding the outcome of patients with severe aortic stenosis after chest radiation therapy?

A. Post-procedural atrial fibrillation is more common in transcatheter aortic valve replacement (TAVR) than in surgical aortic valve replacement (SAVR).
B. SAVR is associated with a shorter hospital stay when compared to TAVR.
C. SAVR is associated with a lower adjusted 1-year all-cause mortality when compared to TAVR in this patient population.
D. TAVR is associated with a lower adjusted 30-day all-cause mortality.

40. A 60-year-old male presents to the Cardio-Oncology Clinic for evaluation of an elevated resting heart rate. The patient has history of Hodgkin's lymphoma treated with thoracic radiation therapy and anthracycline-containing chemotherapy 20 years ago. Which of the following statements is correct regarding previous treatment with thoracic radiation and the development of autonomic dysfunction?

A. Abnormal heart rate recovery predicts increased all-cause mortality in survivors treated with thoracic radiation therapy.
B. Autonomic dysfunction is associated with the presence of cardiovascular risk factors.
C. Autonomic dysfunction is characterized by increased parasympathetic and attenuated sympathetic activity.
D. Prevalence of autonomic dysfunction is independent of time from thoracic radiation therapy.

41. Which of the following interventions is associated with a significant reduction in stroke in patients treated with radiation therapy to the head, neck, and thorax?

A. Atorvastatin
B. Fish oil
C. Lisinopril
D. Metoprolol

42. A 45-year-old female with hormone-receptor-positive breast cancer is started on adjuvant endocrine therapy. Which of the following is most accurate regarding the risk of venous thromboembolism (VTE) among breast cancer survivors treated with adjuvant endocrine therapy?

A. Both tamoxifen and aromatase inhibitors have a similar risk of VTE.
B. Tamoxifen is associated with a higher risk of VTE compared to an aromatase inhibitor.
C. Aromatase inhibitors are associated with a higher VTE risk than tamoxifen.
D. There is no increased risk of VTE.

43. Among patients with prostate cancer and high baseline cardiovascular (CV) risk, prolonged exposure (more than 6 months) to androgen deprivation therapy (ADT) has been associated with:

A. Good cardiorespiratory fitness (CRF), but reduced CV mortality
B. Good CRF and paradoxical increased CV mortality
C. Reduced CRF and increased CV mortality
D. Reduced CRF and no significant effect on CV mortality

44. What is the recommended duration of anticoagulation for the treatment of cancer-associated venous thromboembolic disease?

A. At least 1 month
B. At least 3 months
C. At least 6 months
D. At least 12 months

45. There are several proposed mechanisms responsible for the significant hypertensive response seen with vascular endothelial growth factor (VEGF) inhibitors. Which of the following is the most accurate explanation for this effect?

A. A functional increase in nitric oxide production
B. A reduction in endothelin-1 activity
C. A substantial increase in vascular resistance and left ventricular afterload
D. An increase in capillary density as that seen in anatomic rarefaction

46. A 64-year-old female with metastatic breast cancer presents with worsening shortness of breath. A chest X-ray shows an enlarged cardiac silhouette. A transthoracic echocardiogram shows a large, circumferential pericardial effusion with

indeterminate hemodynamic measurements for tamponade. Physical examination shows an elevated jugular venous pressure. What is the best next step?

A. Obtain a cardiac magnetic resonance imaging (MRI) with gadolinium contrast
B. Perform a pericardiocentesis and send sample for cytology
C. Perform a right and left heart catheterization
D. Repeat a transthoracic echocardiogram in 6 weeks

47. A 65-year-old male with stable coronary artery disease is treated with cabozantinib for renal cell carcinoma. He is also on aspirin 81 mg daily and atorvastatin 80 mg daily. During his follow up appointment, his blood pressure is 160/86 mmHg. He denied having any symptoms. Of the following, what is the best way to manage his hypertension?

A. Begin an angiotensin-converting enzyme (ACE) inhibitor and continue cabozantinib
B. Begin diltiazem and continue cabozantinib without interruption
C. Begin verapamil, hold cabozantinib and resume when the blood pressure is within normal range
D. Stop cabozantinib and consider a different treatment for renal cell carcinoma

48. Immune checkpoint blocking antibodies increase anti-tumor immunity by:

A. Activating normal co-inhibitory molecules on T cells
B. Activating normal co-stimulatory molecules on T cells
C. Inhibiting normal co-inhibitory molecules on T cells
D. Inhibiting normal co-stimulatory molecules on T cells

49. Which of the following is a potential complication seen in patients with acute promyelocytic leukemia treated with all-trans retinoic acid and/or arsenic trioxide?

A. Differentiation syndrome
B. Hemophagocytic lymphohistiocytosis (HLH)
C. Macrophage activation syndrome
D. Trousseau syndrome

50. Which of the following screening biomarkers has been shown to have both diagnostic and prognostic significance for cardiac involvement in patients with carcinoid heart disease?

A. Activin A
B. Cardiac troponin T
C. Chromogranin A
D. N-terminal pro-B-type natriuretic peptide (NT-proBNP)

51. A 48-year-old female with metastatic neuroendocrine intestinal tumor is being evaluated for liver transplantation. She has New York Heart Association class 3 symptoms and a heart failure hospitalization in the past 6 months. Transthoracic echocardiogram showed mild right ventricular hypertrophy, thickened and restricted tricuspid valve leaflets that failed to coapt, severe tricuspid regurgitation, and evidence of a thickened pulmonary valve with severe regurgitation. The patient is currently on furosemide, spironolactone, and octreotide. What is the best next step in the cardiovascular management of this patient?

A. Proceed with liver transplantation and repeat an echocardiogram in 6 months
B. Referral for heart transplantation prior to liver transplantation
C. Tricuspid and pulmonary valve replacement prior to liver transplantation
D. Tricuspid valve replacement prior to liver transplantation

52. Which of the following statements is correct about carriers of clonal hematopoiesis of indeterminate potential (CHIP)?

A. CHIP confers a 40% increase in cardiovascular risk.
B. Individuals with CHIP have a 5% increase in all-cause mortality.
C. The diagnosis of CHIP requires the presence of definitive morphological evidence of a hematologic neoplasm.
D. The risk of developing a hematologic malignancy is greater than 1% per year.

53. A 35-year-old female with history of childhood Hodgkin's lymphoma presents to her follow-up appointment for chronic systolic heart failure due to chemotherapy-induced cardiomyopathy (CCMP). Her left ventricular ejection fraction is 20% and she continues to experience New York Heart Association class 4 symptoms. Which of the following statements is most accurate in patients with CCMP undergoing heart transplantation?

A. CCMP patients are more likely to require biventricular support before heart transplantation than patients with other non-ischemic cardiomyopathies.
B. CCMP patients have worse survival after heart transplantation than patients with other non-ischemic cardiomyopathies.
C. CCMP patients tend to have more co-morbidities compared to other non-ischemic cardiomyopathy patients.
D. The incidence of infection after heart transplantation is similar to other patients.

54. A 65-year-old female with leiomyosarcoma of the uterus is diagnosed with acute deep vein thrombosis (DVT) of the right lower extremity. She has completed 7 months of anticoagulation with rivaroxaban 20 mg daily without complications. A month ago, she started to notice swelling in the left lower extremity while on rivaroxaban. An ultrasound shows a new DVT in that extremity. What is the best next step in the management of DVT in this patient?

A. Change to warfarin
B. Change to low-molecular-weight heparin
C. Continue rivaroxaban for at least 6 more months
D. Insert a vena cava filter

55. Which of the following statements is most accurate about the long-term use of a vena cava filter in the management of venous thromboembolism (VTE) in patients with cancer?

A. A permanent filter is preferred in patients with cancer.
B. It has been shown to decrease the risk of pulmonary embolism.
C. It improves survival.
D. It is associated with an increased long-term risk for lower extremity thrombus.

56. Which of the following criteria are the principal determinants defining the severity of cytokine release syndrome?

A. Fever and arthralgia
B. Fever and coagulopathy
C. Hypotension and hypoxia
D. Pleural effusion and tachycardia

57. A 68-year-old female with uterine cancer presents with worsening left lower extremity swelling and tenderness over the past 2 weeks. There is evidence of skin ulceration and venous engorgement. A venous ultrasound shows an acute thrombus in the common femoral vein. What is the best next step in the management of this patient?

A. Initiate dabigatran and repeat a venous ultrasound in 3 months
B. Initiate aspirin and warfarin and repeat a venous ultrasound in 3 months
C. Initiate low-molecular-weight heparin and consider percutaneous mechanical thrombectomy
D. Place an inferior vena cava filter and reassess in 3 months

58. A 59-year-old male with metastatic neuroendocrine tumor with primary involvement of the liver presents with worsening lower extremity edema and pain. The patient had undergone extensive evaluation with multiple venous ultrasounds showing no evidence of deep vein thrombosis. A transthoracic echocardiogram showed normal left ventricular function and no valve disease. N-terminal pro-brain natriuretic peptide (NT-proBNP) is normal. What is the next best step in the management of this patient?

A. Obtain a cardiac MRI
B. Obtain a CT scan with contrast of the chest, abdomen, and pelvis
C. Recommend wearing compression stockings
D. Start furosemide and repeat a venous ultrasound

59. A 57-year-old male with metastatic adenocarcinoma of the esophagus presents with worsening dyspnea on exertion and atrial fibrillation with rapid ventricular response. A transthoracic echocardiogram revealed right ventricular dilation with free wall hypokinesis and apical sparing. A chest CT scan demonstrates extensive bilateral pulmonary emboli and a large thrombus within the right atrium. Blood pressure is 90/50 mmHg and heart rate is 110 beats per minute. In addition to starting anticoagulation, what is the next best step to consider in the management of this patient?

    A. Cardiac catheterization with coronary angiogram
    B. Evaluate for thrombectomy
    C. Systemic thrombolysis
    D. Transesophageal echocardiogram and possible direct-current cardioversion

60. A 70-year-old female presents with worsening fatigue and dyspnea on exertion. She was diagnosed with desmoid fibromatosis and was started on sorafenib. She has history of Hodgkin lymphoma 30 years ago treated with non-anthracycline containing chemotherapy and no radiation therapy per patient's wishes. She has history of mitral valve disease requiring replacement with a bioprosthetic valve one year ago. Vital signs in clinic showed a pulse of 61 beats per minute (bpm), blood pressure of 120/60 mmHg, respiratory rate of 12 breaths per minute, and oxygen saturation on room air of 99%. Physical examination revealed an irregularly irregular rhythm, holosystolic murmur at the left lower sternal border, and normal jugular venous pressure. Electrocardiogram demonstrated atrial fibrillation with a heart rate of 60 bpm. What is the best next step in the management of this patient?

    A. Dobutamine stress echocardiogram
    B. Cardiac catheterization with coronary angiography
    C. Transesophageal echocardiogram with possible direct-current cardioversion
    D. Transthoracic echocardiogram with Doppler

61. A 25-year-old male with history of Hodgkin's lymphoma at the age of 12 years was referred for cardiovascular surveillance. His cancer treatment included four cycles of ABVE (doxorubicin with cumulative dose of 200 mg/m^2, bleomycin, vincristine, and etoposide) and mantle radiation. He denies having any symptoms at this time and his vital signs are within normal range. A thyroid ultrasound showed a right-sided 2-centimeter solid, hypoechoic nodule. Fine-needle aspiration demonstrated atypia of undetermined significance. What is the best next step in the management of this patient?

    A. Perform a PET-CT scan
    B. Referral for hemithyroidectomy for excision
    C. Repeat a thyroid ultrasound in 12 months
    D. Repeat a thyroid ultrasound in 6 months

62. A 61-year-old male with chronic systolic heart failure with a left ventricular ejection fraction less than 20% and normal right ventricular size and function has been diagnosed with prostate adenocarcinoma (Gleason grade 3+4 = 7 on the right and Gleason grade 4+3 = 7 on the left). His most recent prostate-specific antigen (PSA) is 80 ng/mL, previously 40 ng/mL two months ago. Bone scintigraphy shows no evidence of osseous metastatic disease. He is now admitted for the fourth time with acute on chronic systolic heart failure requiring inotropic therapy with dobutamine. What is the best next step in the management of this patient?

    A. Discharge home on palliative dobutamine
    B. Referral for heart transplantation
    C. Referral for left ventricular assist device and start prostate cancer therapy
    D. Referral to hospice

63. A 60-year-old male with a large right hilar/suprahilar pulmonary mass invading the mediastinum presents with recurrent headaches and swelling of the face and upper extremities. Vital signs showed a pulse of 108 beats per minute (bpm), blood pressure of 89/55 mmHg, respiratory rate of 16 breaths per minute, and oxygen saturation on room air 98%. What is the most likely diagnosis?

    A. Acute coronary syndrome
    B. Acute pulmonary embolism
    C. Cardiac tamponade
    D. Superior vena cava syndrome

64. What is the most appropriate therapeutic intervention to address the diagnosis in Question 63?

    A. Endovascular recanalization with or without stenting
    B. High-dose intravenous steroids
    C. Radiation therapy
    D. Systemic thrombolytic therapy

65. A 67-year-old male with essential hypertension and asymptomatic paroxysmal atrial fibrillation is diagnosed with mantle cell lymphoma. In addition to easy bruising, he also has intermittent nausea. His oncologist recommends treatment with ibrutinib. Due to the potential for drug-drug interaction, which of the following medications should be avoided when a patient is taking ibrutinib?

    A. Amlodipine
    B. Diltiazem
    C. Metoprolol
    D. Prochlorperazine (Compazine)

66. A 72-year-old female is enrolled in a clinical trial evaluating a novel oral tyrosine kinase inhibitor for the treatment of advanced thyroid cancer. Pre-clinical studies suggested a possible impact on cardiac repolarization. Which of the following statements is correct regarding QT interval evaluation in patients undergoing cancer treatment?

    A. QT interval prolongation is a more significant issue with arsenic trioxide than with nilotinib.
    B. QT interval prolongation is rarely associated with oral cancer therapies.
    C. The Bazett formula is the preferred correction formula for oncology patients.
    D. Ventricular arrhythmias occur in greater than 10% of individuals with significant QT interval prolongation.

67. A 46-year-old female presents to clinic complaining of dyspnea on exertion and new lower extremity edema. She has gained 15 pounds (6.8 kilograms) over the past 3 weeks. Physical examination revealed an elevated jugular venous pressure, ascites, and 2+ bilateral lower extremity pitting edema. A limited, point-of-care echocardiogram showed a normal left ventricular systolic function. Her medical history includes prior Hodgkin lymphoma at the age of 14 years and treatment with mantle radiation. Which of the following test would be most helpful in establishing a diagnosis?

    A. Cardiac magnetic resonance imaging (CMRI)
    B. Contrast-enhanced echocardiography
    C. Nuclear multigated acquisition scan (MUGA)
    D. Transesophageal echocardiogram

68. A 56-year-old male with history of essential hypertension and mixed hyperlipidemia is about to start an anthracycline-based chemotherapy regimen. Which of the following imaging modalities is the most appropriate initial choice for assessing left ventricular function?

    A. Cardiac magnetic resonance imaging (MRI)
    B. Echocardiogram with strain imaging
    C. Nuclear multi-gated acquisition scan (MUGA)
    D. Nuclear stress test

69. Which of the following statements is correct about patients undergoing hematopoietic stem cell transplantation (HSCT)?

    A. Cyclophosphamide can cause significant cardiac morbidity in the acute setting
    B. HSCT is associated with a high prevalence of cardiac mortality
    C. HSCT is rarely associated with volume overload
    D. Late cardiotoxicity from cyclophosphamide is related to cumulative dose

70. A 55-year-old male with multivessel coronary artery disease and severe mitral regurgitation will be undergoing coronary bypass grafting and mitral valve repair. He has been on bevacizumab and FOLFOX (folinic acid, 5-fluorouracil, and oxaliplatin) for 3 months for colon cancer. What would be a reason to delay surgery?

    A. Impaired platelet function
    B. Poor wound healing
    C. Recurrent ischemia with anesthesia
    D. Risk of hypertensive crisis

71. A 55-year-old male presents with acute dyspnea and hypertensive urgency (186/122 mmHg). Blood pressure upon standing was 110/70 mmHg. What test would most likely be diagnostic?

    A. Serum free light chains
    B. Renal ultrasound
    C. Serum catecholamines
    D. Urine 5 HIAA

72. A 26-year-old female is seen by her obstetrician for a second trimester visit. A mass is discovered in her right breast and biopsy shows inflammatory breast cancer. Which of the following is a true statement regarding breast cancer and pregnancy?

    A. Chemotherapy increases the risk of early delivery
    B. Chemotherapy is safe during all trimesters
    C. Pregnancy should be terminated
    D. Breast surgery is her only option

73. A 45-year-old male with AML (acute myelogenous leukemia) achieves remission after 7+3 induction (cytarabine and idarubicin). He complains of almost disabling positional lightheadedness. On exam, supine blood pressure is 100/74 mmHg and standing blood pressure is 68/44 mmHg. Serum electrolytes are within normal range. What is the most likely cause of his orthostatic hypotension?

    A. Adrenal insufficiency
    B. Anthracycline cardiac toxicity
    C. Cytarabine cardiac toxicity
    D. Immune-mediated autonomic dysfunction

74. Which of the following favors that a cardiac mass is malignant on a cardiac MRI?

    A. Abnormal first pass perfusion
    B. Left atrial location
    C. Narrow base of attachment
    D. Size 2-3 cm

75. Which of the following is true of imaging cardiac tumors?

A. 3D echocardiography is superior to 2D echocardiography in assessing size
B. A high carbohydrate diet is required to adequately evaluate cardiac tumors by FDG PET
C. Microscopic calcification is best determined by cardiac MRI
D. Use of ultrasound enhancing agent is FDA-approved to evaluate tumor perfusion

76. In which clinical condition is cardiac MRI preferred over echocardiography?

A. 5-fluorouracil associated acute coronary syndrome
B. Cardiac tamponade
C. Radiation-induced valvular heart disease
D. Suspected myocarditis

77. A 62-year-old male with acute myeloid leukemia (AML) achieves remission after induction with 7+3 (cytarabine and idarubicin) and consolidation with HiDAC (high dose cytarabine). He undergoes a 10/10 matched unrelated donor allogeneic stem cell transplantation. His serum creatinine is 0.9 mg/dL, potassium 3.4 mmol/L, and magnesium 1.2 mg/dL. On day 12 post-stem cell transplant, he has the following electrocardiogram (ECG). The most likely cause of this ECG abnormality is:

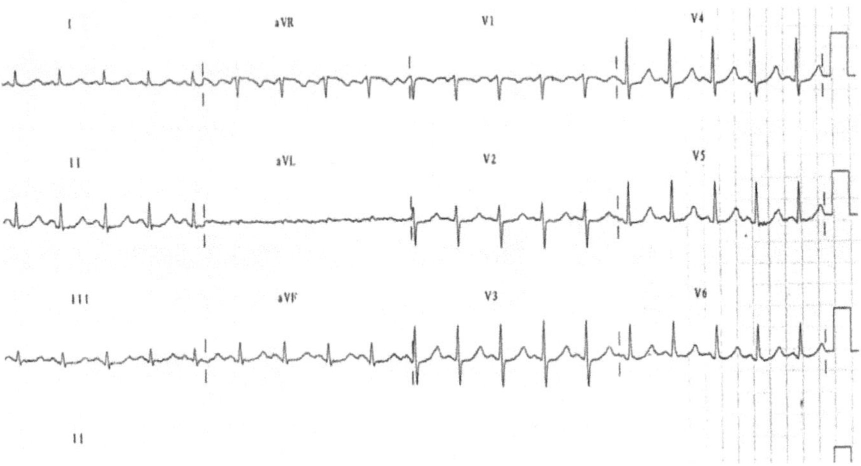

A. Acyclovir
B. Letermovir
C. Prednisone
D. Tacrolimus

78. A 47-year-old female is diagnosed with stage IV non-Hodgkin lymphoma with a high tumor burden. On day 5 of her treatment, she complains of nausea, vomiting, and palpitations. The nurse notices that her urine is "dark". Which of the following would you expect to see in checking her electrolytes?

A. Hypercalcemia
B. Hyperphosphatemia
C. Hypokalemia
D. Hypouricemia

79. A 49-year-old female who is 11 months post orthotopic renal transplant presents with new onset of fever and dyspnea. She has a bulky mediastinal mass on chest imaging. A biopsy of the mass is consistent with CD20+ post-transplant lymphoproliferative disease (PTLD). What is the most effective treatment for her?

A. Allogeneic stem cell transplantation
B. Everolimus
C. Mediastinal radiation
D. Rituximab

80. A 23-year-old male with sickle cell disease is admitted with a vaso-occlusive crisis and anemia. On exam, his temperature is 99 degrees Fahrenheit, blood pressure is 124/75 mmHg, and pulse is 110 beats per minute. His oxygen saturation on room air is 98%. He is transfused 2 units of packed red blood cells (PRBCs) for worsening anemia. At the end of his second unit of PRBCs, he reports shortness of breath. Physical examination reveals diffuse bilateral crackles, jugular venous distention, and an S3 on cardiac auscultation. A chest X-ray shows diffuse bilateral infiltrates. What is the most likely diagnosis?

A. Acute chest syndrome
B. Acute pulmonary embolism
C. Transfusion associated circulatory overload (TACO)
D. Transfusion related acute lung injury (TRALI)

81. Which of the following statements is true regarding patients with thalassemia?

A. Cardiac iron overload with heart failure can be successfully reversed with aggressive chelation therapy.
B. Cardiovascular complications are rarely a cause of death in transfusion-dependent thalassemia patients.
C. Sildenafil has been shown to have no benefit in thalassemia patients who develop pulmonary hypertension.
D. There is no role for screening asymptomatic thalassemia patients with normal left ventricular function for iron overload using cardiac magnetic resonance imaging.

82. A 70-year-old male with acute myeloid leukemia (ALL) is currently receiving treatment with venetoclax. He is currently on amlodipine, carvedilol, and lisinopril for essential hypertension and rosuvastatin for mixed hyperlipidemia. Which of his current medications has the potential for significant drug-drug interaction with his cancer therapy?

    A. Amlodipine
    B. Carvedilol
    C. Lisinopril
    D. Rosuvastatin

83. A 35-year-old male with history of Hodgkin lymphoma treated with radiation therapy and ABVD (doxorubicin, bleomycin, vincristine, and dacarbazine) 15 years ago would like to know if he has any sports restrictions. Which of the following sports could be associated with a higher risk of cardiopulmonary complications in this patient?

    A. Baseball
    B. Scuba diving
    C. Soccer
    D. Swimming

84. What is the principal role of the cardio-oncologist during cancer treatment?

    A. Apply target doses of evidence-based heart failure medications
    B. Maintain left ventricular ejection fraction within normal range
    C. Monitor imaging and blood markers of cardiotoxicity
    D. Support safe continuation of cancer therapy

85. Which of the following statements best describes the long-term risk of cardiotoxicity from anthracyclines in childhood cancer survivors?

    A. Dexrazoxane reduces the risk of cardiotoxicity when administered before each dose of doxorubicin.
    B. Doxorubicin given by continuous infusion is no safer than bolus therapy.
    C. Mitoxantrone is associated with a lower risk of cardiotoxicity when compared to doxorubicin.
    D. Surveillance for cardiac dysfunction should be performed more frequently if treatment was given after puberty.

86. Which of the following tyrosine kinase inhibitor (TKI) causes significant hyperlipidemia?

    A. Alectinib
    B. Brigatinib
    C. Lorlatinib
    D. Ponatinib

87. Certain cancer therapeutics can cause hypertriglyceridemia. Which of the following drugs is least likely to significantly elevate serum triglycerides?

A. Anastrozole
B. Asparaginase
C. Baroxotine
D. Capecitabine

88. Which of the following is the most accurate statement regarding radiation therapy for breast cancer?

A. Deep-inspiration breath holding during treatment minimizes cardiac exposure
B. Doubling the number of radiation fractions reduces the risk of toxicity
C. One single high dose treatment is effective treatment and eliminates cardiac toxicity
D. There is no difference in late cardiac toxicity between left and right sided breast cancer treatment

89. Which of the following is correct about anthracycline-associated cardiac toxicity?

A. If there is no overt cardiac toxicity at 10 years after treatment completion, there is no further risk
B. The risk of cardiac toxicity is less with hematologic compared to solid malignancies
C. Topoisomerase II-ß has been implicated
D. Toxicity never occurs when the cumulative dose is less than 100 mg/m^2

90. A 48-year-old female with history of Hodgkin lymphoma at the age of 17 years was treated with mantle radiation. She was recently diagnosed with metastatic ovarian carcinoma and has received one cycle of gemcitabine and cisplatin. She complains of pleuritic anterior chest pain and has a pericardial friction rub on exam. What is the most likely cause of her symptoms?

A. Acute pulmonary embolism
B. Coronary artery spasm
C. Metastatic disease to the lungs
D. Radiation recall

91. Which of the following is a contraindication to radiation therapy in breast cancer?

A. Active scleroderma with vasculitis
B. Diffusing capacity of the lungs for carbon monoxide (DLCO) 90% of the predicted value
C. Presence of a cardiac pacemaker
D. Prior radiation therapy for endometrial carcinoma

92. Which of the following drugs is a cyclin-dependent kinase (CDK) 4/6 inhibitor associated with QT interval prolongation?

    A. Nilotinib
    B. Palbociclib
    C. Ribociclib
    D. Temozolomide

93. A 68-year-old male being treated for mantle cell lymphoma complains of palpitations and lightheadedness. A 24-hour Holter monitor reveals a 15-beat run of monomorphic ventricular tachycardia. Which of the following cancer therapeutics is the most likely cause of his arrhythmia?

    A. Doxorubicin
    B. Fludarabine
    C. Ibrutinib
    D. Rituximab

94. A 45-year-old female with metastatic melanoma is started on combination therapy with dabrafenib and trametinib. Which of the following is the most likely cardiovascular complication with this therapy?

    A. Cardiomyopathy
    B. Hypertension
    C. Pleural effusion
    D. QT interval prolongation

95. Which of the following drugs used in the treatment of T315I-positive chronic myeloid leukemia is associated with arterial and venous thromboembolic events?

    A. Bevacizumab
    B. Osimertinib
    C. Ponatinib
    D. Ruxolitinib

96. Which of the following drugs used in the treatment of metastatic, epidermal growth factor receptor (EGFR) T790M mutation-positive, non-small cell lung cancer is associated with QT interval prolongation and cardiomyopathy?

    A. Afatinib
    B. Dacomitinib
    C. Erlotinib
    D. Osimertinib

97. Which of the following types of cancer is associated with non-bacterial thrombotic endocarditis?

    A. Glioblastoma multiforme
    B. Lymphoma
    C. Melanoma
    D. Pancreas

98. A 65-year-old male with Philadelphia chromosome-positive acute lymphoblastic leukemia on treatment presents with worsening dyspnea on exertion. A chest XR shows a new right-sided pleural effusion and an enlarged cardiac silhouette. Which of the following cancer therapeutics would explain his clinical presentation?

    A. Dasatinib
    B. Imatinib
    C. Nilotinib
    D. Ponatinib

99. Which of the following drugs is an FLT-3 inhibitor associated with QT interval prolongation approved for the treatment of adult patients who have relapsed or refractory acute myeloid leukemia (AML)?

    A. Cabozantinib
    B. Dabrafenib
    C. Gilteritinib
    D. Sorafenib

100. A 67-year-old male with history of hypertension and asymptomatic paroxysmal atrial fibrillation is diagnosed with mantle cell lymphoma. In addition to easy bruising, he also has intermittent nausea resulting from his malignancy. His oncologist recommends starting ibrutinib. Within two weeks of starting ibrutinib, the patient develops symptomatic atrial fibrillation with rapid ventricular response. Considering potential drug-drug interaction, which of the following medications would be most appropriate to manage his atrial fibrillation?

    A. Amiodarone
    B. Diltiazem
    C. Dronedarone
    D. Metoprolol

Answers & Explanations

1. A 45-year-old male with essential hypertension presents with fatigue and exertional dyspnea. He was diagnosed with nodular sclerosis Hodgkin lymphoma at the age of 16 years and achieved his first remission after 6 cycles of ABVD (Adriamycin [doxorubicin], 300 mg/m^2; bleomycin, 120 units/m^2; vinblastine, 72 mg/m^2; and dacarbazine, 4.5 g/m^2), followed by 4000 centigray (cGy) mediastinal radiation. The patient relapsed after 6 months, received ICE (ifosfamide, cyclophosphamide, and etoposide), and subsequently underwent autologous stem cell transplantation. He then achieved complete remission. Which of the following elements of the patient's history are associated with the greatest long-term risk of heart failure?

   A. Bleomycin, dacarbazine

   B. Doxorubicin, mediastinal radiation

   C. Gender, autologous stem cell transplantation

   D. Vinblastine, age 45 years

   The Childhood Cancer Survivor Study (CCSS) consisted of 13,060 childhood survivors who were free of significant cardiovascular disease 5 years after cancer diagnosis. The participants of this study were observed through age 40 years for the development of heart failure. Approximately 37% of individuals received an anthracycline, whereas 26% received chest radiotherapy, excluding scatter <5 Gy. Heart failure risk increased by factors of 1.6, 3.1, and 10.5, following mean heart doses of 5-14 Gy, 15-34 Gy, and ≥35 Gy, respectively, compared with patients who did not have any cardiac radiation exposure. Heart failure risk was also found to increase by factors of 2.1, 3.7, and 10.5 for cumulative anthracycline doses of <100, 100-249, and ≥250 mg/m^2 compared with those not exposed to anthracyclines.

   A case-control study including 2,617 five-year survivors of Hodgkin lymphoma (HL) diagnosed before age 51 years during 1965 to 1995 was conducted to determine the radiation dose-response relationship for heart failure in long-term survivors of adolescent and adult HL, to estimate cumulative risk of heart failure after radiotherapy given with and without anthracyclines, and to assess other determinants of heart failure risk. The authors estimated the mean heart dose and mean left ventricular doses (MLVD) by reconstruction of individual treatments on representative computed tomography datasets. Twenty-five-year cumulative risks of heart failure following MLVDs of 0-15 Gy, 16-20 Gy, and ≥21 Gy were 4.4%, 6.2%, and 13.3%, respectively, in patients treated without anthracycline-containing chemotherapy, and 11.2%, 15.9%, and 32.9%, respectively, in patients treated with anthracyclines. Anthracycline-containing chemotherapy increased heart failure rate, approximately threefold, irrespective of cardiac radiation exposure.

Reference(s):

- Chow EJ, Chen Y, Kremer LC, Breslow NE, Hudson MM, Armstrong GT, Border WL, Feijen EA, Green DM, Meacham LR, Meeske KA, Mulrooney DA, Ness KK, Oeffinger KC, Sklar CA, Stovall M, van der Pal HJ, Weathers RE, Robison LL, Yasui Y. Individual prediction of heart failure among childhood cancer survivors.

J Clin Oncol. 2015 Feb 10;33(5):394-402. doi: 10.1200/JCO.2014.56.1373. Epub 2014 Oct 6. PMID: 25287823; PMCID: PMC4314592.

- van Nimwegen FA, Ntentas G, Darby SC, Schaapveld M, Hauptmann M, Lugtenburg PJ, Janus CPM, Daniels L, van Leeuwen FE, Cutter DJ, Aleman BMP. Risk of heart failure in survivors of Hodgkin lymphoma: effects of cardiac exposure to radiation and anthracyclines. Blood. 2017 Apr 20;129(16):2257-2265. doi: 10.1182/blood-2016-09-740332. Epub 2017 Jan 31. PMID: 28143884; PMCID: PMC5418626.

2. Cytokine release syndrome (CRS) can occur after chimeric antigen receptor-T cell (CAR-T) treatment. Which of the following is a correct statement?

   A. A significant decrease in LVEF (left ventricular ejection fraction) can occur with any grade of CRS.

   B. Pre-existing treatment with anthracyclines is a contraindication to CAR-T therapy.

   C. Troponin level does not correlate with the severity of CRS.

   D. When CRS occurs, the early use of tocilizumab is associated with a lower rate of cardiovascular events.

   A retrospective cohort study including 137 patients who received CAR-T therapy between January 1, 2016 and November 10, 2018 showed that the duration between CRS and tocilizumab administration was associated with cardiovascular events. This risk increased 1.7-fold with each 12-hour delay to tocilizumab. CRS of any grade was common and occurred a median of 5 days after CAR-T therapy: CRS grade ≥2 occurred in 39% of the patients and grade ≥3 in 4%. Among the cohort of 137 patients, only 53 had pre- and post- CAR-T troponin measure, of which 29 of 53 had an increase in troponin after CAR-T administration. When stratified based on CRS grade, 50% of the patients with CRS grade ≥3 had elevated troponin versus 20% among patients with no CRS or grade ≤2. Furthermore, a cardiovascular event occurred in 16 of 29 patients (55%) with an elevated troponin versus 1 of 24 (4.1%) of patients with no elevation of troponin post-CAR-T administration ($p < 0.001$).

Reference(s):

- Alvi RM, Frigault MJ, Fradley MG, Jain MD, Mahmood SS, Awadalla M, Lee DH, Zlotoff DA, Zhang L, Drobni ZD, Hassan MZO, Bassily E, Rhea I, Ismail-Khan R, Mulligan CP, Banerji D, Lazaryan A, Shah BD, Rokicki A, Raje N, Chavez JC, Abramson J, Locke FL, Neilan TG. Cardiovascular Events Among Adults Treated With Chimeric Antigen Receptor T-Cells (CAR-T). J Am Coll Cardiol. 2019 Dec 24;74(25):3099-3108. doi: 10.1016/j.jacc.2019.10.038. PMID: 31856966; PMCID: PMC6938409.

3. A 64-year-old male with history of Philadelphia chromosome positive acute lymphoblastic leukemia undergoes allogeneic hematopoietic stem cell transplantation. His conditioning included busulfan and cyclophosphamide. Post-transplant, he is started on dasatinib maintenance therapy. In addition, he is receiving immunosuppression with tacrolimus. He missed two appointments

for his blood work. He now presents with shortness of breath, tremors, lower extremity edema, worsening hypertension, and acute kidney injury with a serum creatinine of 2.5 mg/dL (previously 0.7 mg/dL). There are shistocytes on peripheral smear review and there is a new reduction in his platelet count. What drug is the most likely cause of his presentation?

A. Busulfan
B. Cyclophosphamide
C. Dasatinib
D. Tacrolimus

Cyclosporine A (CyA) and tacrolimus are calcineurin inhibitors used in the prevention of solid organ transplant rejection and graft-versus-host disease in allogeneic hematopoietic stem cell transplantation. This patient is receiving tacrolimus and has not had surveillance laboratory tests on 2 occasions. His clinical presentation is suggestive of tacrolimus toxicity and thrombotic microangiopathy. CyA and tacrolimus toxicity has been studied extensively in renal transplantation, and it is now recognized that CyA renal toxicity can present in different ways: acute reversible decrease in glomerular filtration rate, acute microvascular disease with the pattern of thrombotic microangiopathy, and chronic irreversible renal damage. Other potential adverse effects relevant to the cardio-oncology patient include hypertension, arrhythmias, new onset diabetes mellitus after transplant, electrolyte abnormalities, hyperlipidemia, hypertriglyceridemia, and weight gain. Patients receiving tacrolimus and other immunosuppressive agents require close surveillance.

Reference(s):

- Araya AA, Tasnif Y. Tacrolimus. [Updated 2020 Jun 9]. In: StatPearls [Internet]. Treasure Island (FL): StatPearls Publishing; 2021 Jan-. Available from: https://www.ncbi.nlm.nih.gov/books/NBK544318/
- Remuzzi G, Bertani T. Renal vascular and thrombotic effects of cyclosporine. Am J Kidney Dis. 1989 Apr;13(4):261-72. doi: 10.1016/s0272-6386(89)80032-0. PMID: 2650537.

4. Which of the following cardiac abnormalities carries the highest risk in the Hematopoietic Cell Transplantation-Specific Comorbidity Index?

A. Arrhythmia
B. Congestive heart failure
C. Coronary artery disease
D. Valvular disease (except asymptomatic mitral valve prolapse)

In an effort to better predict outcomes in patients undergoing hematopoietic stem cell transplantation (HCT), Dr. Mohamed Sorror and his team at the University of Washington conducted a study that was designed to better define previously identified comorbidities using pre-transplant laboratory data, investigate additional HCT-related comorbidities, and establish comorbidity scores that were suited for HCT. The HCT-specific comorbidity index is depicted on the following table.

Comorbidity	Definition of comorbidities	Scores
History of arrhythmia	Atrial fibrillation or flutter, sick sinus syndrome, or ventricular arrhythmias	1
Cardiac disease	Coronary artery disease (≥1 vessel coronary stenosis requiring medical treatment, stent, or bypass graft), heart failure with reduced (EF ≤50%) or preserved ejection fraction, myocardial infarction	1
Valvular heart disease	Except mitral valve prolapse	3
Inflammatory bowel disease	Crohn disease or ulcerative colitis	1
Diabetes	Requiring treatment with insulin or oral therapy but not diet alone	1
Cerebrovascular disease	Transient ischemic attack or cerebrovascular accident	1
Psychiatric disturbance	Depression or anxiety requiring psychiatric consult or treatment	1
Mild hepatic disease	Chronic hepatitis, bilirubin > upper limit of normal (ULN) to 1.5 times ULN, or AST/ALT > ULN to 2.5 times ULN	1
Moderate/ severe hepatic disease	Liver cirrhosis, bilirubin >1.5 times ULN, or AST/ALT >2.5 ULN	3
Obesity	Body mass index >35 kg/m^2	1
Infection	Requiring continuation of antimicrobial treatment after day 0	1
Rheumatologic	Systemic lupus erythematosus, rheumatoid arthritis, polymyositis, mixed connective tissue disease, or poly-myalgia rheumatic	2
Peptic ulcer disease	Requiring treatment	2
Moderate/ severe renal disease	Serum creatinine >2 mg/dL, on dialysis, or prior renal transplantation	2
Prior solid tumor	Treated at any time point in the patient's past history, excluding non-melanoma skin cancer	3
Moderate pul-monary disease	DL_{CO} and/or FEV_1 66-80% or dyspnea on slight activity	2
Severe pulmo-nary disease	DL_{CO} and/or FEV_1 ≤65% or dyspnea at rest or requir-ing oxygen	3

Reference(s):

- Sorror ML, Maris MB, Storb R, Baron F, Sandmaier BM, Maloney DG, Storer B. Hematopoietic cell transplantation (HCT)-specific comorbidity index: a new tool for risk assessment before allogeneic HCT. Blood. 2005 Oct 15;106(8):2912-9. doi: 10.1182/blood-2005-05-2004. Epub 2005 Jun 30. PMID: 15994282; PMCID: PMC1895304.

5. All of the following statements are correct regarding Chimeric Antigen Receptor (CAR) T-cell therapy, EXCEPT:

   A. Life-threatening hemodynamic instability and cardiogenic shock is usually attributed to Cytokine Release Syndrome (CRS) after CAR T-cell therapy.

   B. Multiple studies have shown that cardiovascular manifestations of CRS are due to off-target cross-reactivity of T-cell receptors against the striated muscle-specific protein.

   C. Routine monitoring of NT-proBNP or BNP level in patients receiving CAR T-cell therapy helps identify patients for early tocilizumab administration

   D. Steroids are routinely given to prevent the development of CRS after CAR T-cell therapy.

   According to the 2020 Society for Immunotherapy of Cancer (SITC) clinical practice guideline on immune effector cell-related adverse events, the panel recommends the following management strategies:

- For elderly patients or patients with extensive comorbidities, tocilizumab should be considered earlier in the course of CRS.
- For adults who develop American Society for Transplantation and Cellular Therapy (ASTCT) grade 2 CRS, tocilizumab may be considered.
- In both adults and children, if CRS does not improve after 1 dose of tocilizumab, then steroids should be administered with a second dose of tocilizumab.
- If CRS does not improve after 2 doses of tocilizumab (and steroids), third-line agents, including anakinra, siltuximab, and high-dose methylprednisolone should be considered.
- If CRS does not improve after tocilizumab and steroids, infections should be considered again in the differential diagnosis and managed appropriately.
- If steroids are used in the management of CRS, a rapid taper should be used once symptoms begin to improve.

In a recent study including 100 patients with relapsed or refractory large B-cell lymphoma treated with standard of care anti-CD19 CAR T-cell therapy, higher cumulative dose of corticosteroids and prolonged and early use after CAR T-cell infusion were associated with shorter progression-free survival and overall survival, respectively. According to the authors, corticosteroids should be used at the lower dose and for the shortest duration. The initiation of corticosteroids should also be delayed whenever clinically possible.

Reference(s):

- Maus MV, Alexander S, Bishop MR, Brudno JN, Callahan C, Davila ML, Diamonte C, Dietrich J, Fitzgerald JC, Frigault MJ, Fry TJ, Holter-Chakrabarty JL, Komanduri KV, Lee DW, Locke FL, Maude SL, McCarthy PL, Mead E, Neelapu SS, Neilan TG, Santomasso BD, Shpall EJ, Teachey DT, Turtle CJ, Whitehead T, Grupp SA. Society for Immunotherapy of Cancer (SITC) clinical practice guideline on immune effector cell-related adverse events. J Immunother Cancer. 2020 Dec;8(2):e001511. doi: 10.1136/jitc-2020-001511. PMID: 33335028; PMCID: PMC7745688.
- Strati P, Ahmed S, Furqan F, Fayad LE, Lee HJ, Iyer SP, Nair R, Nastoupil LJ, Parmar S, Rodriguez MA, Samaniego F, Steiner RE, Wang M, Pinnix CC, Horowitz SB, Feng L, Sun R, Claussen CM, Hawkins MC, Johnson NA, Singh P, Mistry H, Johncy S, Adkins S, Kebriaei P, Shpall EJ, Green MR, Flowers CR, Westin J, Neelapu SS. Prognostic impact of corticosteroids on efficacy of chimeric antigen receptor T-cell therapy in large B-cell lymphoma. Blood. 2021 Jun 10;137(23):3272-3276. doi: 10.1182/blood.2020008865. PMID: 33534891; PMCID: PMC8351896.

6. Which of the following statements is true regarding cardiac tumors?

   A. Cardiac rhabdomyosarcoma is the most common primary cardiac tumor in adults.

   B. Compared to metastatic cardiac tumors, primary cardiac tumors are more common.

   C. Primary cardiac masses are most commonly found in the right atrium and pericardium.

   D. The majority of primary cardiac tumors are malignant.

   Although cardiac tumors are rare, they can be associated with significant morbidity and mortality. Based on 12,485 consecutive autopsies performed in a 20-year period between 1972 and 1991 at Queen Mary Hospital in Hong Kong, the autopsy incidence of primary and secondary cardiac tumors was 0.056% and 1.23%, respectively. In another study that included 8,069 consecutive patients referred for cardiac MRI between May 2008 and August 2013, 145 (1.8%) had a cardiac mass. Among 53 cases that had histological correlation, 25 (47%) were benign, 26 (49%) were metastatic, and 2 (4%) were malignant primary cardiac masses. The most common locations were intracavitary masses (39%) with the right atrium being the most common chamber (21%), followed by extrapericardial masses with cardiac extension (20%).

Reference(s):

- Lam KY, Dickens P, Chan AC. Tumors of the heart. A 20-year experience with a review of 12,485 consecutive autopsies. Arch Pathol Lab Med. 1993 Oct;117(10):1027-31. PMID: 8215825.

- Maleszewski JJ, Bois MC, Bois JP, Young PM, Stulak JM, Klarich KW. Neoplasia and the Heart: Pathological Review of Effects With Clinical and Radiological Correlation. J Am Coll Cardiol. 2018 Jul 10;72(2):202-227. doi: 10.1016/j.jacc.2018.05.026. PMID: 29976295.
- Mousavi N, Cheezum MK, Aghayev A, Padera R, Vita T, Steigner M, Hulten E, Bittencourt MS, Dorbala S, Di Carli MF, Kwong RY, Dunne R, Blankstein R. Assessment of Cardiac Masses by Cardiac Magnetic Resonance Imaging: Histological Correlation and Clinical Outcomes. J Am Heart Assoc. 2019 Jan 8;8(1):e007829. doi: 10.1161/JAHA.117.007829. PMID: 30616453; PMCID: PMC6405700.

7. Which of the following malignancies rarely metastasizes to the heart?

   A. Breast cancer

   B. Lung cancer

   C. Melanoma

   D. Prostate cancer

   Malignancies can affect the heart by different mechanisms: direct extension, hematogenous spread, retrograde lymphatic seeding, and venous extension. The likelihood of cardiac involvement by a tumor depends on the stage of disease and individual tumor and patient's biology. The most common malignancies to involve the heart are lung cancer, breast cancer, hematologic malignancies (lymphomas, leukemias), and melanoma. Other cancers with high rates of cardiac involvement include ovarian, gastric, renal, and pancreatic malignancies as well as mesothelioma. Prostate cancer rarely metastasizes to the heart.

Reference(s):

- Bussani R, De-Giorgio F, Abbate A, Silvestri F. Cardiac metastases. J Clin Pathol. 2007 Jan;60(1):27-34. doi: 10.1136/jcp.2005.035105. Epub 2006 Nov 10. PMID: 17098886; PMCID: PMC1860601.
- Goldberg AD, Blankstein R, Padera RF. Tumors metastatic to the heart. Circulation. 2013 Oct 15;128(16):1790-4. doi: 10.1161/CIRCULATIONAHA.112.000790. PMID: 24126323.
- Maleszewski JJ, Bois MC, Bois JP, Young PM, Stulak JM, Klarich KW. Neoplasia and the Heart: Pathological Review of Effects With Clinical and Radiological Correlation. J Am Coll Cardiol. 2018 Jul 10;72(2):202-227. doi: 10.1016/j.jacc.2018.05.026. PMID: 29976295.

8. Which of the following syndromes is associated with cardiac myxomas?

   A. Carney complex

   B. Gorlin syndrome

   C. Li-Fraumeni syndrome

   D. Tuberous sclerosis

Carney complex is a rare autosomal dominant syndrome caused by inactivating mutations or large deletions of the PRKAR1A gene located at 17q22-24 coding for the regulatory protein subunit type I alpha of protein kinase A (PKA) gene). It is characterized by pigmented lesions of the skin and mucosa, cardiac, cutaneous, and other myxomas and multiple endocrine tumors. Cardiac myxomas are the most common non-cutaneous lesions found in Carney complex and can be found anywhere in the heart and equally present in males and females. In contrast, sporadic cardiac myxomas have a predilection for the left atrium and are more common in older female patients.

Gorlin syndrome, also known as nevoid basal cell carcinoma syndrome, is an autosomal dominant syndrome associated with a mutation in the tumor suppressor gene PATCHED. The typical clinical triad is characterized by multiple basal cell carcinoma, keratocystic odontogenic tumors, and cerebral calcifications. The diagnosis of this syndrome is based on major and minor clinical criteria. Major imaging-based criteria include the presence of keratocystic odontogenic tumors of the jaw before the age of 20 years, lamellar calcifications of the falx cerebri, and medulloblastoma. Other major criteria include a first-degree relative with Gorlin syndrome, multiple basal cell carcinoma (more than expected by the degree of sun damage received) or one in a patient younger than 20 years of age. Minor imaging-based criteria include rib abnormalities (bified, fused, splayed), ovarian or cardiac fibroma, lymphomesenteric cysts, macrocephaly, and skeletal abnormalities (e.g., Sprengel deformity, pectus, kyphoscoliosis). Other minor criteria include ocular abnormalities (cataracts, glaucoma) and congenital anomalies such as cleft lip and hypertelorism.

Tuberous sclerosis is an autosomal dominant syndrome caused by mutations in the tumor suppressor genes tuberous sclerosis complex 1 (TSC1/hamartin) and tuberous sclerosis complex 2 (TSC2/tuberin). This syndrome is associated with cardiac rhabdomyomas, which can be found in up to 50% of patients.

Li-Fraumeni syndrome is a rare hereditary condition characterized by germline TP53 mutations resulting in the development of cancers in multiple organ systems. It is not typically associated with cardiac tumors and specifically, with cardiac myxomas.

Reference(s):

- Correa R, Salpea P, Stratakis CA. Carney complex: an update. Eur J Endocrinol. 2015 Oct;173(4):M85-97. doi: 10.1530/EJE-15-0209. Epub 2015 Jun 30. PMID: 26130139; PMCID: PMC4553126.
- Espiard S, Bertherat J. Carney complex. Front Horm Res. 2013;41:50-62. doi: 10.1159/000345669. Epub 2013 Mar 19. PMID: 23652670.
- Lee E, Mahani MG, Lu JC, Dorfman AL, Srinivasan A, Agarwal PP. Primary cardiac tumors associated with genetic syndromes: a comprehensive review. PediatrRadiol. 2018 Feb;48(2):156-164. doi: 10.1007/s00247-017-4027-2. Epub 2017 Dec 6. PMID: 29214333.

McBride KA, Ballinger ML, Killick E, Kirk J, Tattersall MH, Eeles RA, Thomas DM, Mitchell G. Li-Fraumeni syndrome: cancer risk assessment and clinical management. Nat Rev Clin Oncol. 2014 May;11(5):260-71. doi: 10.1038/nrclinonc.2014.41. Epub 2014 Mar 18. PMID: 24642672.

9. Which of the findings below, in the setting of high clinical suspicion for amyloid cardiomyopathy, is most specific for AL (light chain) amyloidosis?

   A. Interventricular septum measuring >1.2 centimeters (cm)

   B. Carpal tunnel syndrome

   C. Macroglossia

   D. Prominent cardiac uptake on pyrophosphate scan

   Approximately 10% of patients with AL amyloidosis have macroglossia, which may vary from tongue enlargement to subtle tooth indentation of the tongue.

Reference(s):

- Falk RH, Alexander KM, Liao R, Dorbala S. AL (Light-Chain) Cardiac Amyloidosis: A Review of Diagnosis and Therapy. J Am Coll Cardiol. 2016 Sep 20;68(12):1323-41. doi: 10.1016/j.jacc.2016.06.053. PMID: 27634125.

10. Based on the Childhood Cancer Survivor Study (CCSS), childhood cancer survivors are at increased risk for heart failure, coronary artery disease, pericardial disease, and valvular disease. Which of the following factors has been shown to have a statistically significant association with all of these cardiovascular events?

    A. Doxorubicin therapy with a cumulative dose greater than 250 mg/m^2

    B. History of lymphoma

    C. Radiotherapy dose

    D. Younger age at diagnosis (before the age of 10 years)

    A retrospective cohort study was conducted to investigate the impact of modifications to contemporary cancer protocols on serious cardiac outcomes among adult survivors of childhood cancer. The study consisted of 23,462 participants in the Childhood Cancer Survivor Study (CCSS) of which 6,193 were treated in the 1970s, 9,363 in the 1980s, and 7,906 in the 1990s. They were all diagnosed with one of the following malignancies—leukemia, brain cancer, Hodgkin lymphoma, non-Hodgkin lymphoma, renal tumors, neuroblastoma, soft tissue sarcomas, and bone sarcomas—before the age of 21 years between January 1, 1970 and December 31, 1999. Risk factors for heart failure, coronary artery disease, pericardial disease, and valvular heart disease are listed below. It is important to recognize that compared with survivors with a diagnosis of malignancy in the 1970s, the risk of heart failure, coronary artery disease, and valvular heart disease decreased in the 1980s and 1990s, but only significantly for coronary artery disease. The overall risk of coronary artery disease was reduced by adjustment for cardiac radiation, especially among survivors of Hodgkin lymphoma.

Heart failure	Coronary artery disease	Pericardial disease	Valvular heart disease
■ Female sex ■ Higher mean heart radiation dose ■ Higher cumulative dose of anthracycline ■ Diabetes ■ Dyslipidemia ■ Hypertension	■ Higher mean heart radiation dose ■ Dyslipidemia ■ Hypertension	■ Higher mean radiation dose ■ Hypertension	■ Higher mean heart radiation dose ■ Hypertension

Reference(s):

- Mulrooney DA, Hyun G, Ness KK, Ehrhardt MJ, Yasui Y, Duprez D, Howell RM, Leisenring WM, Constine LS, Tonorezos E, Gibson TM, Robison LL, Oeffinger KC, Hudson MM, Armstrong GT. Major cardiac events for adult survivors of childhood cancer diagnosed between 1970 and 1999: report from the Childhood Cancer Survivor Study cohort. BMJ. 2020 Jan 15;368:l6794. doi: 10.1136/bmj.l6794. PMID: 31941657; PMCID: PMC7190022.

11. A 29-year-old female presents with acute systolic heart failure and atrial fibrillation. Upon further questioning, the patient informed us that she was treated for Hodgkin lymphoma as a child. Which of the following may have contributed to the patient's current condition?

    A. Cisplatin

    B. Cyclophosphamide

    C. Dacarbazine

    D. Doxorubicin

    The most common multiagent chemotherapy regimens are MOPP (mechlorethamine, vincristine, procarbazine, and prednisone) and ABVD (doxorubicin, bleomycin, vinblastine, and dacarbazine). In general, MOPP-related sequelae include dose-related risk of infertility and the development of myelodysplasia and leukemia. ABVD is associated with a higher risk of cardiopulmonary toxicity due to doxorubicin and bleomycin. All of the agents in the original MOPP and ABVD regimens continue to be used in contemporary pediatric treatment regimens.

Name	Drugs	References
ABVD	Doxorubicin, bleomycin, vinblastine, dacarbazine	■ Bonadonna G, Santoro A. ABVD chemotherapy in the treatment of Hodgkin's disease. Cancer Treat Rev. 1982;9(1):21-35. doi:10.1016/s0305-7372(82)80003-0 ■ Mefferd JM, Donaldson SS, Link MP. Pediatric Hodgkin's disease: pulmonary, cardiac, and thyroid function following combined modality therapy. Int J Radiat Oncol Biol Phys. 1989;16(3):679-685. doi:10.1016/0360-3016(89)90485-9 ■ Weiner MA, Leventhal BG, Marcus R, et al. Intensive chemotherapy and low-dose radiotherapy for the treatment of advanced-stage Hodgkin's disease in pediatric patients: a Pediatric Oncology Group study. J Clin Oncol. 1991;9(9):1591-1598. doi:10.1200/JCO.1991.9.9.1591
ABVE-PC	Doxorubicin, bleomycin, vincristine, etoposide, prednisone, cyclophosphamide	■ Schwartz CL, Constine LS, Villaluna D, et al. A risk-adapted, response-based approach using ABVE-PC for children and adolescents with intermediate- and high-risk Hodgkin lymphoma: the results of P9425 [published correction appears in Blood. 2016 Jul 28;128(4):605]. Blood. 2009;114(10):2051-2059. doi:10.1182/blood-2008-10-184143
AV-PC	Doxorubicin, vincristine, prednisone, cyclophosphamide	■ Appel BE, Chen L, Buxton AB, et al. Minimal Treatment of Low-Risk, Pediatric Lymphocyte-Predominant Hodgkin Lymphoma: A Report From the Children's Oncology Group. J Clin Oncol. 2016;34(20):2372-2379. doi:10.1200/JCO.2015.65.3469

Name	Drugs	References
		■ Keller FG, Castellino SM, Chen L, et al. Results of the AHOD0431 trial of response adapted therapy and a salvage strategy for limited stage, classical Hodgkin lymphoma: A report from the Children's Oncology Group. Cancer. 2018;124(15):3210-3219. doi:10.1002/cncr.31519
BEACOPP	Bleomycin, etoposide, doxorubicin, cyclophosphamide, vincristine, prednisone, procarbazine	■ Kelly KM, Sposto R, Hutchinson R, et al. BEACOPP chemotherapy is a highly effective regimen in children and adolescents with high-risk Hodgkin lymphoma: a report from the Children's Oncology Group. Blood. 2011;117(9):2596-2603. doi:10.1182/blood-2010-05-285379
COPDAC	Dacarbazine (substituted for procarbazine in COPP)	■ Mauz-Körholz C, Hasenclever D, Dörffel W, et al. Procarbazine-free OEPA-COPDAC chemotherapy in boys and standard OPPA-COPP in girls have comparable effectiveness in pediatric Hodgkin's lymphoma: the GPOH-HD-2002 study. J Clin Oncol. 2010;28(23):3680-3686. doi:10.1200/JCO.2009.26.9381
COPP	Cyclophosphamide, vincristine, procarbazine, prednisone	■ Mauz-Körholz C, Hasenclever D, Dörffel W, et al. Procarbazine-free OEPA-COPDAC chemotherapy in boys and standard OPPA-COPP in girls have comparable effectiveness in pediatric Hodgkin's lymphoma: the GPOH-HD-2002 study. J Clin Oncol. 2010;28(23):3680-3686. doi:10.1200/JCO.2009.26.9381
COPP/ABV	Cyclophosphamide, vincristine, procarbazine, prednisone, doxorubicin, bleomycin, vinblastine	■ Weiner MA, Leventhal BG, Marcus R, et al. Intensive chemotherapy and low-dose radiotherapy for the treatment of advanced-stage Hodgkin's disease in pediatric patients: a Pediatric Oncology Group study. J Clin Oncol. 1991;9(9):1591-1598. doi:10.1200/JCO.1991.9.9.1591

Name	Drugs	References
CVP	Cyclophosphamide, vinblastine, prednisone	■ Shankar A, Hall GW, Gorde-Grosjean S, et al. Treatment outcome after low intensity chemotherapy [CVP] in children and adolescents with early stage nodular lymphocyte predominant Hodgkin's lymphoma - an Anglo-French collaborative report. Eur J Cancer. 2012;48(11):1700-1706. doi:10.1016/j.ejca.2011.10.018
DBVE	Doxorubicin, bleomycin, vincristine, etoposide	■ Tebbi CK, Mendenhall N, London WB, et al. Treatment of stage I, IIA, IIIA1 pediatric Hodgkin disease with doxorubicin, bleomycin, vincristine and etoposide (DBVE) and radiation: a Pediatric Oncology Group (POG) study. Pediatr Blood Cancer. 2006;46(2):198-202. doi:10.1002/pbc.20546 ■ Tebbi CK, Mendenhall NP, London WB, et al. Response-dependent and reduced treatment in lower risk Hodgkin lymphoma in children and adolescents, results of P9426: a report from the Children's Oncology Group. Pediatr Blood Cancer. 2012;59(7):1259-1265. doi:10.1002/pbc.24279
MOPP	Mechlorethamine, vincristine, procarbazine, and prednisone	■ Donaldson SS, Link MP. Combined modality treatment with low-dose radiation and MOPP chemotherapy for children with Hodgkin's disease. J Clin Oncol. 1987;5(5):742-749. doi:10.1200/JCO.1987.5.5.742 ■ Devita VT Jr, Serpick AA, Carbone PP. Combination chemotherapy in the treatment of advanced Hodgkin's disease. Ann Intern Med. 1970;73(6):881-895. doi:10.7326/0003-4819-73-6-881

Name	Drugs	References
		■ Ortin TT, Shostak CA, Donaldson SS. Gonadal status and reproductive function following treatment for Hodgkin's disease in childhood: the Stanford experience. Int J Radiat Oncol Biol Phys. 1990;19(4):873-880. doi:10.1016/0360-3016(90)90007-7
OEPA	Vincristine, etoposide, prednisone, doxorubicin	■ Mauz-Körholz C, Hasenclever D, Dörffel W, et al. Procarbazine-free OEPA-COPDAC chemotherapy in boys and standard OPPA-COPP in girls have comparable effectiveness in pediatric Hodgkin's lymphoma: the GPOH-HD-2002 study. J Clin Oncol. 2010;28(23):3680-3686. doi:10.1200/JCO.2009.26.9381
OPPA	Vincristine, procarbazine, prednisone, doxorubicin	■ Mauz-Körholz C, Hasenclever D, Dörffel W, et al. Procarbazine-free OEPA-COPDAC chemotherapy in boys and standard OPPA-COPP in girls have comparable effectiveness in pediatric Hodgkin's lymphoma: the GPOH-HD-2002 study. J Clin Oncol. 2010;28(23):3680-3686. doi:10.1200/JCO.2009.26.9381
VAMP	Vinblastine, doxorubicin, methotrexate, prednisone	■ Donaldson SS, Link MP, Weinstein HJ, et al. Final results of a prospective clinical trial with VAMP and low-dose involved-field radiation for children with low-risk Hodgkin's disease. J Clin Oncol. 2007;25(3):332-337. doi:10.1200/JCO.2006.08.4772

Other Reference(s):

- PDQ Pediatric Treatment Editorial Board. Childhood Hodgkin Lymphoma Treatment (PDQ®): Health Professional Version. In: PDQ Cancer Information Summaries. Bethesda (MD): National Cancer Institute (US); June 21, 2021.

12. Anthracycline use has been associated with significant cardiac dysfunction. Which of the following treatments has been shown to be effective at primary prevention of cardiac dysfunction?

    A. Carvedilol

    B. Dexrazoxane

    C. Enalapril

    D. Sacubitril-valsartan

    Anthracyclines are well known to cause cardiac toxicity in a dose-dependent manner. Dexrazoxane prevents mitochondrial destruction by binding to iron and prevention the formation of superhydroxide radicals.

    In a phase II single-arm non-inferiority trial in patients with metastatic or unresectable soft-tissue sarcoma treated with a median dose of doxorubicin of 450 mg/m², upfront use of dexrazoxane was associated with a progression-free survival of 8.4 months (95% confidence interval: 5.1-11.2 months), no cardiac hospitalizations, and no new, persistent cardiac dysfunction with left ventricular ejection fraction less than 50%. Only 3 patients were removed from this study due to cardiotoxicity and had received >600 mg/m² of doxorubicin.

Reference(s):

- Seifert CF, Nesser ME, Thompson DF. Dexrazoxane in the prevention of doxorubicin-induced cardiotoxicity. Ann Pharmacother. 1994 Sep;28(9):1063-72. doi: 10.1177/106002809402800912. Erratum in: Ann Pharmacother 1994 Dec;28(12):1413. PMID: 7803884.
- Van Tine BA, Hirbe AC, Oppelt P, Frith AE, Rathore R, Mitchell JD, Wan F, Berry S, Landeau M, Heberton GA, Gorcsan J 3rd, Huntjens PR, Soyama Y, Vader JM, Alvarez-Cardona JA, Zhang KW, Lenihan DJ, Krone RJ. Interim Analysis of the Phase II Study: Noninferiority Study of Doxorubicin with Upfront Dexrazoxane plus Olaratumab for Advanced or Metastatic Soft-Tissue Sarcoma. Clin Cancer Res. 2021 Jul 15;27(14):3854-3860. doi: 10.1158/1078-0432.CCR-20-4621. Epub 2021 Mar 25. PMID: 33766818; PMCID: PMC8282681.

13. A 26-year-old male with history of Hodgkin lymphoma at the age of 12 years was referred to the Cardio-Oncology Clinic for cardiovascular surveillance. He was treated with 4 courses of ABVE (doxorubicin [cumulative dose 200 mg/m²], bleomycin, vincristine, and etoposide) in addition to mantle field radiation therapy. The patient is asymptomatic. He has stage 2 hypertension. A lipid panel demonstrates an elevated LDL 146 mg/dL (3.78 mmol/L). His body mass index is 28 kg/m² and has no family history of cardiovascular disease. Carotid Doppler ultrasound demonstrates mild atherosclerotic disease of the right external carotid artery. In addition to lifestyle modification, which of the following is the best treatment option for this patient?

    A. Observation and reassess his blood pressure and lipid panel in 3-6 months

    B. Start fish oil and pharmacologic antihypertensive therapy

    C. Start pharmacologic antihypertensive therapy and niacin

    D. Start pharmacologic antihypertensive therapy and statin therapy

This is a young patient with premature atherosclerotic disease affecting his carotid artery. His risk factors for atherosclerosis and the development of a cardiovascular event include history of mantle field radiation therapy, uncontrolled essential hypertension, and hypercholesterolemia. According to the 2018 Guideline on the Management of Blood Cholesterol, this patient has evidence of atherosclerotic cardiovascular disease and would benefit from lifestyle modification plus high-intensity statin aiming to reduce his low-density lipoprotein (LDL) cholesterol by ≥50% (Class I recommendation). If high-intensity statin is not tolerated, a moderate-intensity statin should be used (Class I recommendation). If after a period on maximal stain therapy the LDL-C remains ≥70 mg/dL (≥1.8 mmol/L), adding ezetimibe may be reasonable (Class IIb recommendation).

According to the 2017 High Blood Pressure Clinical Practice Guideline, a patient's blood pressure should be classified based on the following categories.

Category	Systolic Blood Pressure (SBP)		Diastolic Blood Pressure (DBP)
Normal	<120 mmHg	and	<80 mmHg
Elevated	120-129 mmHg	and	<80 mmHg
Hypertension			
Stage 1	130-139 mmHg	and/or	80-89 mmHg
Stage 2	≥140 mmHg	and/or	≥90 mmHg

This patient has stage 2 hypertension with evidence of atherosclerotic cardiovascular disease. In addition, he has history of mantle field radiation therapy and is at risk for renal parenchymal disease and renovascular disease. The use of blood pressure-lowering medications is recommended for secondary prevention of recurrent cardiovascular events in patients with clinical cardiovascular disease and an average systolic blood pressure (SBP) ≥130 mmHg or an average diastolic blood pressure (DBP) ≥80 mmHg, and for primary prevention in adults with an estimated 10-year atherosclerotic cardiovascular disease (ASCVD) risk ≥10% and an average SBP ≥130 mmHg or an average DBP ≥80 mmHg (Class I recommendation). Moreover, for patients with no history of cardiovascular disease and an estimated 10-year ASCVD risk <10% but with an SBP ≥140 mmHg or a DBP ≥90 mmHg, the use of blood pressure-lowering medications is recommended for primary prevention of cardiovascular disease (Class I recommendation). This is in addition to lifestyle changes.

Reference(s):

- Grundy SM, Stone NJ, Bailey AL, Beam C, Birtcher KK, Blumenthal RS, Braun LT, de Ferranti S, Faiella-Tommasino J, Forman DE, Goldberg R, Heidenreich PA, Hlatky MA, Jones DW, Lloyd-Jones D, Lopez-Pajares N, Ndumele CE, Orringer CE, Peralta CA, Saseen JJ, Smith SC Jr, Sperling L, Virani SS, Yeboah J. 2018 AHA/ACC/AACVPR/AAPA/ABC/ACPM/ADA/AGS/APhA/ASPC/NLA/PCNA Guideline on the Management of Blood Cholesterol: A Report of the American College of Cardiology/American Heart Association Task Force on

Clinical Practice Guidelines. Circulation. 2019 Jun 18;139(25):e1082-e1143. doi: 10.1161/CIR.0000000000000625. Epub 2018 Nov 10. Erratum in: Circulation. 2019 Jun 18;139(25):e1182-e1186. PMID: 30586774.

- Whelton PK, Carey RM, Aronow WS, Casey DE Jr, Collins KJ, Dennison Himmelfarb C, DePalma SM, Gidding S, Jamerson KA, Jones DW, MacLaughlin EJ, Muntner P, Ovbiagele B, Smith SC Jr, Spencer CC, Stafford RS, Taler SJ, Thomas RJ, Williams KA Sr, Williamson JD, Wright JT Jr. 2017 ACC/AHA/AAPA/ABC/ACPM/AGS/APhA/ASH/ASPC/NMA/PCNA Guideline for the Prevention, Detection, Evaluation, and Management of High Blood Pressure in Adults: A Report of the American College of Cardiology/American Heart Association Task Force on Clinical Practice Guidelines. J Am Coll Cardiol. 2018 May 15;71(19):e127-e248. doi: 10.1016/j.jacc.2017.11.006. Epub 2017 Nov 13. Erratum in: J Am Coll Cardiol. 2018 May 15;71(19):2275-2279. PMID: 29146535.

14. A 69-year-old female with metastatic invasive ductal carcinoma of the right breast was referred to the Cardio-Oncology clinic before starting trastuzumab. Five years ago, she received anthracycline-based therapy for triple negative (HER2 negative, estrogen receptor negative, and progesterone receptor negative) breast cancer. One year after anthracycline therapy she developed mild symptomatic heart failure with a left ventricular ejection fraction (LVEF) of 38% and was started on enalapril and carvedilol. A new transthoracic echocardiogram reveals a non-dilated left ventricle with LVEF of 49%. The patient is asymptomatic (NYHA class 1 symptoms). Which of the following statements is true regarding the use of trastuzumab in this patient?

    A. Invasive coronary angiography should be performed prior to initiating trastuzumab.

    B. She can start trastuzumab since she has a low risk of developing cardiac dysfunction.

    C. The patient can be started on trastuzumab with close cardiac safety monitoring.

    D. Trastuzumab is contraindicated.

    Nowsheen et al performed a retrospective study of women treated with trastuzumab for HER2 positive breast cancer at Mayo Clinic Rochester between January 1, 2000 and August 31, 2015. Their study demonstrated that women undergoing trastuzumab therapy with impaired baseline cardiac function (20/428 women had a baseline left ventricular ejection fraction [LVEF] 45.4±7% before trastuzumab) experienced no higher risk of LVEF decline, but more frequently developed symptomatic heart failure. Initiation or intensification of cardioprotective medications with or without transient or permanent discontinuation of trastuzumab was associated with a smaller fraction of patients with irreversible decline in LVEF to <20%. Due to a higher cardiac risk in this population, these patients should be followed and co-managed by a cardio-oncologist.

    The SAFE-HEaRt study was a pilot study assessing the cardiac safety of trastuzumab, pertuzumab, and T-DM1 in patients with stage I-IV HER2-positive breast cancer with cardiac dysfunction at baseline (LVEF 40-49%) and no heart failure symptoms. Fifteen patients were treated with trastuzumab, 14 with trastuzumab and pertuzumab, and 2 with TDM-1. The mean LVEF was 45% at baseline and 46% at the end of treatment. Three patients experienced a cardiac event (defined as heart failure, myocardial infarction, arrhythmia, cardiac death, or significant asymptomatic worsening of LVEF). The authors concluded that HER2-targeted therapies were safe in patients with reduced cardiac function (LVEF 40-49%) and concomitant treatment with carvedilol and renin angiotensin inhibitors, highlighting the importance of a collaborative approach between cardio-oncologists and oncologists in the care of these patients.

References:

- Lynce F, Barac A, Geng X, Dang C, Yu AF, Smith KL, Gallagher C, Pohlmann PR, Nunes R, Herbolsheimer P, Warren R, Srichai MB, Hofmeyer M, Cunningham A, Timothee P, Asch FM, Shajahan-Haq A, Tan MT, Isaacs C, Swain SM. Prospective evaluation of the cardiac safety of HER2-targeted therapies in patients with HER2-positive breast cancer and compromised heart function: the SAFE-HEaRt study. Breast Cancer Res Treat. 2019 Jun;175(3):595-603. doi: 10.1007/s10549-019-05191-2. Epub 2019 Mar 9. PMID: 30852761; PMCID: PMC6534513.
- Nowsheen S, Aziz K, Park JY, Lerman A, Villarraga HR, Ruddy KJ, Herrmann J. Trastuzumab in Female Breast Cancer Patients With Reduced Left Ventricular Ejection Fraction. J Am Heart Assoc. 2018 Aug 7;7(15):e008637. doi: 10.1161/JAHA.118.008637. PMID: 30371238; PMCID: PMC6201446.

15. A 56-year-old male with melanoma presents with palpitations and chest pain. He was started on pembrolizumab 4 weeks ago. Transthoracic echocardiogram showed a normal left ventricular ejection fraction. Cardiac troponin is mildly elevated. Electrocardiogram was unremarkable. What would be the best next diagnostic test?

    A. Cardiac magnetic resonance imaging (MRI)

    B. Dobutamine stress echocardiogram

    C. Endomyocardial biopsy

    D. Transesophageal echocardiogram

    Recognition of immune checkpoint inhibitor (ICI)-related myocarditis is of utmost importance because it is associated with a significantly higher mortality when compared to other immune-related adverse events. Clinical presentation may vary and a high level of suspicion is often warranted. The ideal diagnostic test is one that confirms the diagnosis of myocarditis while excluding other more common causes of the clinical manifestations presented in this case such as acute coronary syndrome. Cardiac MRI is the non-invasive imaging modality of choice to diagnose myocarditis. Although endomyocardial biopsy is considered the gold standard diagnostic test for myocarditis, it has technical limitations as in the case of focal or patchy myocarditis. In addition, this may not be readily available in many centers and requires a pathologist with experience in this area.

Reference(s):

- Ferreira VM, Schulz-Menger J, Holmvang G, Kramer CM, Carbone I, Sechtem U, Kindermann I, Gutberlet M, Cooper LT, Liu P, Friedrich MG. Cardiovascular Magnetic Resonance in Nonischemic Myocardial Inflammation: Expert Recommendations. J Am Coll Cardiol. 2018 Dec 18;72(24):3158-3176. doi: 10.1016/j.jacc.2018.09.072. PMID: 30545455.
- Palaskas N, Lopez-Mattei J, Durand JB, Iliescu C, Deswal A. Immune Checkpoint Inhibitor Myocarditis: Pathophysiological Characteristics, Diagnosis, and Treatment. J Am Heart Assoc. 2020 Jan 21;9(2):e013757. doi: 10.1161/JAHA.119.013757. Epub 2020 Jan 21. PMID: 31960755; PMCID: PMC7033840.

16. A 58-year-old female with history of hypertension and diabetes is currently receiving doxorubicin for breast cancer. Her baseline echocardiogram shows a normal left ventricular ejection fraction (LVEF) of 63% and global longitudinal strain (GLS) of -21%. An echocardiogram was obtained after the patient presented with shortness of breath and it showed a decrease in LVEF to 56% and GLS to -15%. Select the correct statement regarding the observed reduction in GLS.

    A. A reduction in GLS during treatment has no clinical significance if the LVEF remains normal.

    B. A reduction in GLS from -21% to -15.0% is indicative of subclinical LV dysfunction.

    C. GLS decline >25% correlates with a reduction in LVEF at 1 year.

    D. Temporarily hold cancer treatment until GLS improves

    The patient's left ventricular GLS decreased from -21% to -15%, which represents a 29% relative drop in GLS. According to the 2014 Expert Consensus for Multimodality Imaging Evaluation of Adult Patients during and after Cancer Therapy, a relative drop in GLS greater than 15% is suggestive of subclinical LV dysfunction.

Reference(s):

- Plana JC, Galderisi M, Barac A, Ewer MS, Ky B, Scherrer-Crosbie M, Ganame J, Sebag IA, Agler DA, Badano LP, Banchs J, Cardinale D, Carver J, Cerqueira M, DeCara JM, Edvardsen T, Flamm SD, Force T, Griffin BP, Jerusalem G, Liu JE, Magalhães A, Marwick T, Sanchez LY, Sicari R, Villarraga HR, Lancellotti P. Expert consensus for multimodality imaging evaluation of adult patients during and after cancer therapy: a report from the American Society of Echocardiography and the European Association of Cardiovascular Imaging. J Am Soc Echocardiogr. 2014 Sep;27(9):911-39. doi: 10.1016/j.echo.2014.07.012. PMID: 25172399.

17. Which of the following modalities is preferred if 2-dimensional transthoracic echocardiography provides inaccurate or discrepant measurements of left ventricular systolic function due to poor image quality?

A. Cardiac magnetic resonance imaging (MRI)
B. Contrast-enhanced gated cardiac computed tomography (CT)
C. Non-contrast 3-dimensional echocardiography
D. Nuclear multigated acquisition scan (MUGA)

Cardiac MRI is the reference standard in the evaluation of left and right ventricular RV) volumes and left ventricular ejection fraction (LVEF). It also provides information about pericardial and valvular heart disease. Contrast-enhanced cardiac MRI can also provide information about myocardial tissue, specifically the presence of inflammation and/or fibrosis. Although the calculation of LVEF by MUGA is highly reproducible, it exposes the patient to radiation and does not provide relevant information on pericardial and valvular heart disease and RV function. The accuracy and reproducibility of three-dimensional echocardiography depends on image quality. For this reason, this imaging technique would not be recommended when image quality is poor.

Reference(s):

- Plana JC, Galderisi M, Barac A, Ewer MS, Ky B, Scherrer-Crosbie M, Ganame J, Sebag IA, Agler DA, Badano LP, Banchs J, Cardinale D, Carver J, Cerqueira M, DeCara JM, Edvardsen T, Flamm SD, Force T, Griffin BP, Jerusalem G, Liu JE, Magalhães A, Marwick T, Sanchez LY, Sicari R, Villarraga HR, Lancellotti P. Expert consensus for multimodality imaging evaluation of adult patients during and after cancer therapy: a report from the American Society of Echocardiography and the European Association of Cardiovascular Imaging. J Am Soc Echocardiogr. 2014 Sep;27(9):911-39. doi: 10.1016/j.echo.2014.07.012. PMID: 25172399.

18. For a patient receiving trastuzumab and being monitored by echocardiography every 3 months, which of the following scenarios is most suggestive of subclinical left ventricular dysfunction?

A. A relative decrease in GLS by 15% compared to baseline
B. A relative increase in GLS by 15% compared to baseline
C. An absolute decrease in global longitudinal strain (GLS) from -20% to -18%
D. An absolute increase in GLS from -18% to -23%

A recent meta-analysis by Oikonomou et al exploring the prognostic value of GLS for the prediction of cancer therapy-related cardiac dysfunction (CTRCD) showed that among patients with cancer, including breast cancer, hematologic malignancies, or sarcomas, treated with anthracyclines with or without trastuzumab, the incidence of CTRCD ranged from 9.3% to 43.8% over a mean follow-up of 4.2 to 23 months (pooled incidence, 21%). In patients receiving active treatment, the high-risk absolute GLS cut-off values ranged from -21% to -13.8%, with worse GLS associated with a higher CTRCD risk (odds ratio, 12.27%; 95% confidence interval (CI), 7.73-19.47; area under the hierarchical summary receiver operating characteristic curve (HSROC) 0.86; 95% CI, 0.83-0.89). For relative changes versus a baseline value, cut-off values ranged from 2.3% to 15.9%, with a greater decrease linked to a 16-fold higher risk of CRTCD. However, both indices showed significant publication bias. The authors concluded that in this meta-analysis, measurement of GLS after initiation of potentially cardiotoxicity therapy had good prognostic performance for subsequent CTRCD. They also recognized the need for larger prospective multicenter studies to support these findings and provide guidance for application in clinical practice.

In the SUCCOUR trial, 331 anthracycline-treated patients with another heart failure risk factor were randomized to cardioprotective therapy initiation guided by either ≥12% relative reduction in GLS or >10% absolute reduction of left ventricular ejection fraction (LVEF). At 1-year follow-up, there was no significant change in LVEF between the 2 arms, but there was a significantly higher use of cardioprotective therapy, and fewer patients met CTRCD criteria in the GLS-guided than the EF-guided arm (5.8% vs 13.7%; p = 0.02).

Reference(s):

- Oikonomou EK, Kokkinidis DG, Kampaktsis PN, Amir EA, Marwick TH, Gupta D, Thavendiranathan P. Assessment of Prognostic Value of Left Ventricular Global Longitudinal Strain for Early Prediction of Chemotherapy-Induced Cardiotoxicity: A Systematic Review and Meta-analysis. JAMA Cardiol. 2019 Oct 1;4(10):1007-1018. doi: 10.1001/jamacardio.2019.2952. PMID: 31433450; PMCID: PMC6705141.
- Plana JC, Galderisi M, Barac A, Ewer MS, Ky B, Scherrer-Crosbie M, Ganame J, Sebag IA, Agler DA, Badano LP, Banchs J, Cardinale D, Carver J, Cerqueira M, DeCara JM, Edvardsen T, Flamm SD, Force T, Griffin BP, Jerusalem G, Liu JE, Magalhães A, Marwick T, Sanchez LY, Sicari R, Villarraga HR, Lancellotti P. Expert consensus for multimodality imaging evaluation of adult patients during and after cancer therapy: a report from the American Society of Echocardiography and the European Association of Cardiovascular Imaging. J Am Soc Echocardiogr. 2014 Sep;27(9):911-39. doi: 10.1016/j.echo.2014.07.012. PMID: 25172399.
- Thavendiranathan P, Negishi T, Somerset E, Negishi K, Penicka M, Lemieux J, Aakhus S, Miyazaki S, Shirazi M, Galderisi M, Marwick TH; SUCCOUR Investigators. Strain-Guided Management of Potentially Cardiotoxic Cancer Therapy. J Am Coll Cardiol. 2021 Feb 2;77(4):392-401. doi: 10.1016/j.jacc.2020.11.020. Epub 2020 Nov 18. PMID: 33220426.

19. Which of the following statements is true regarding the presence coronary artery calcification in patients with cancer?

    A. A high coronary artery calcium (CAC) score is associated with a lower risk of cardiovascular events in women with breast cancer.

    B. Current guidelines recommend obtaining a CAC score 2 years after thoracic radiotherapy.

    C. The main limitation of the CAC score is the high radiation dose.

    D. The presence of coronary artery calcification on a staging CT scan of the chest can be used to determine cardiovascular risk.

The presence of coronary artery calcification (CAC) on planning CT scans was shown to be associated with cardiovascular disease (CVD), especially coronary artery disease (CAD). This was illustrated in a multicenter cohort study consisting of 15,915 patients with breast cancer receiving radiotherapy between 2005 and 2016. The main outcomes were the occurrence of fatal and nonfatal CVD and CAD. After a median follow-up of approximately 52 months, CVD risks increased from 5.2% in patients with no CAC to 28.2% in patients with CAC scores higher than 400. CAC was strongly associated with CAD, and the association between CAC and CVD was strongest in patients treated with anthracyclines and those who received a radiation boost.

Moreover, the International Cardio-Oncology Society published an expert consensus in which it is recommended to review available CT chest imaging for the presence of coronary and aortic calcification before radiotherapy to improve cardiovascular risk stratification and mitigation of future atherosclerotic cardiovascular events.

Reference(s):

- Gal R, van Velzen SGM, Hooning MJ, Emaus MJ, van der Leij F, Gregorowitsch ML, Blezer ELA, Gernaat SAM, Lessmann N, Sattler MGA, Leiner T, de Jong PA, Teske AJ, Verloop J, Penninkhof JJ, Vaartjes I, Meijer H, van Tol-Geerdink JJ, Pignol JP, van den Bongard DHJG, Išgum I, Verkooijen HM. Identification of Risk of Cardiovascular Disease by Automatic Quantification of Coronary Artery Calcifications on Radiotherapy Planning CT Scans in Patients With Breast Cancer. JAMA Oncol. 2021 Jul 1;7(7):1024-1032. doi: 10.1001/jamaoncol.2021.1144. PMID: 33956083; PMCID: PMC8283560.
- Mitchell JD, Cehic DA, Morgia M, Bergom C, Toohey J, Guerrero PA, Ferencik M, Kikuchi R, Carver JR, Zaha VG, Alvarez-Cardona JA, Szmit S, Daniele AJ, Lopez-Mattei J, Zhang L, Herrmann J, Nohria A, Lenihan DJ, Dent SF. Cardiovascular Manifestations From Therapeutic Radiation: A Multidisciplinary Expert Consensus Statement From the International Cardio-Oncology Society. JACC CardioOncol. 2021 Sep 21;3(3):360-380. doi: 10.1016/j.jaccao.2021.06.003. PMID: 34604797; PMCID: PMC8463721.

20. A 48-year-old female with metastatic non-small cell lung cancer (anaplastic lymphoma kinase [ALK] positive) diagnosed 6 months ago presents to clinic complaining of dizziness and fatigue. Her vital signs revealed a blood pressure 110/60 mmHg, pulse 35 beats per minute (bpm), respiratory rate 10 breaths per minute, afebrile, and oxygen saturation 98% on room air. A 12-lead electrocardiogram demonstrated sinus bradycardia with a heart rate of 33 bpm. Which of the following treatments could potentially explain the patient's current presentation?

    A. Bevacizumab

    B. Crizotinib

    C. Lenvatinib

    D. Osimertinib

Choice B is the correct answer. All other choices are not associated with bradycardia and in the clinical trials leading to the approval of crizotinib, there was a recognized dose adjustment protocol for the frequently observed bradycardia using this drug. A recent review of all oral chemotherapy highlighted this observation.

Reference(s):

- Rao VU, Reeves DJ, Chugh AR, O'Quinn R, Fradley MG, Raghavendra M, Dent S, Barac A, Lenihan D. Clinical Approach to Cardiovascular Toxicity of Oral Antineoplastic Agents: JACC State-of-the-Art Review. J Am Coll Cardiol. 2021 Jun 1;77(21):2693-2716. doi: 10.1016/j.jacc.2021.04.009. PMID: 34045027; PMCID: PMC8091379.

21. A 55-year-old male with chronic lymphocytic leukemia (CLL) is started on ibrutinib. Which of the following best describes its mechanism of action?

    A. BCR-ABL kinase inhibitor
    B. Cyclin-dependent kinase (CDK) inhibitor of CDK4 and 6
    C. JAK tyrosine kinase inhibitor
    D. Small-molecule inhibitor of Bruton's tyrosine kinase

Reference(s):

- Ganatra S, Sharma A, Shah S, Chaudhry GM, Martin DT, Neilan TG, Mahmood SS, Barac A, Groarke JD, Hayek SS, Dani S, Venesy D, Patten R, Nohria A. Ibrutinib-Associated Atrial Fibrillation. JACC Clin Electrophysiol. 2018 Dec;4(12):1491-1500. doi: 10.1016/j.jacep.2018.06.004. Epub 2018 Aug 29. PMID: 30573111.

22. Which of the following is an anti-CD38 monoclonal antibody used to treat multiple myeloma?

    A. Bevacizumab
    B. Carfilzomib
    C. Daratumumab
    D. Rituximab

    The GRIFFIN trial, a phase 2 randomized study, demonstrated that the addition of daratumumab to lenalidomide, bortezomib, and dexamethasone (RVd) for transplant-eligible newly-diagnosed multiple myeloma improved response rates and depth of response, including stringent complete remission and minimal residual disease negativity. These findings are consistent with those demonstrated in CASSIOPEIA, which explored the effect of adding daratumumab to bortezomib, thalidomide, and dexamethasone.

Reference(s):

- Moreau P, Attal M, Hulin C, Arnulf B, Belhadj K, Benboubker L, Béné MC, Broijl A, Caillon H, Caillot D, Corre J, Delforge M, Dejoie T, Doyen C, Facon T, Sonntag C, Fontan J, Garderet L, Jie KS, Karlin L, Kuhnowski F, Lambert J, Leleu X, Lenain P, Macro M, Mathiot C, Orsini-Piocelle F, Perrot A, Stoppa AM, van de Donk NW,

Wuilleme S, Zweegman S, Kolb B, Touzeau C, Roussel M, Tiab M, Marolleau JP, Meuleman N, Vekemans MC, Westerman M, Klein SK, Levin MD, Fermand JP, Escoffre-Barbe M, Eveillard JR, Garidi R, Ahmadi T, Zhuang S, Chiu C, Pei L, de Boer C, Smith E, Deraedt W, Kampfenkel T, Schecter J, Vermeulen J, Avet-Loiseau H, Sonneveld P. Bortezomib, thalidomide, and dexamethasone with or without daratumumab before and after autologous stem-cell transplantation for newly diagnosed multiple myeloma (CASSIOPEIA): a randomised, open-label, phase 3 study. Lancet. 2019 Jul 6;394(10192):29-38. doi: 10.1016/S0140-6736(19)31240-1. Epub 2019 Jun 3. Erratum in: Lancet. 2019 Jun 14;: PMID: 31171419.

- Voorhees PM, Kaufman JL, Laubach J, Sborov DW, Reeves B, Rodriguez C, Chari A, Silbermann R, Costa LJ, Anderson LD Jr, Nathwani N, Shah N, Efebera YA, Holstein SA, Costello C, Jakubowiak A, Wildes TM, Orlowski RZ, Shain KH, Cowan AJ, Murphy S, Lutska Y, Pei H, Ukropec J, Vermeulen J, de Boer C, Hoehn D, Lin TS, Richardson PG. Daratumumab, lenalidomide, bortezomib, and dexamethasone for transplant-eligible newly diagnosed multiple myeloma: the GRIFFIN trial. Blood. 2020 Aug 20;136(8):936-945. doi: 10.1182/blood.2020005288. PMID: 32325490; PMCID: PMC7441167.

23. A 65-year-old male was diagnosed with metastatic prostate cancer and is started on abiraterone. His grandson, who is a medical student, would like to know the drug's mechanism of action and potential adverse effects. Which of the following best describes abiraterone's mechanism of action and cardiovascular adverse effect profile?

    A. A gonadotropin releasing hormone (GnRH) agonist – increased risk of myocardial infarction

    B. A gonadotropin releasing hormone (GnRH) antagonist – QT interval prolongation

    C. An androgen biosynthesis inhibitor – hypertension

    D. An androgen receptor inhibitor – metabolic syndrome

GnRH Agonist	GnRH Antagonist	Androgen Receptor Inhibitor	Androgen Biosynthesis Inhibitor
■ Leuprolide ■ Goserelin ■ Triptorelin	■ Degarelix ■ Relugolix	■ Enzalutamide ■ Apalutamide ■ Darolutamide	■ Abiraterone

Cardiovascular effects of androgen deprivation therapy (incidence may depend on the agent)

- Dyslipidemia
- Sarcopenic obesity
- Insulin resistance, metabolic syndrome, diabetes mellitus
- Hypertension
- Cerebrovascular disease, including transient ischemia attack, stroke
- Coronary artery disease, including myocardial infarction
- QT interval prolongation and sudden cardiac death

Reference(s):

- Boland J, Choi W, Lee M, Lin J. Cardiovascular Toxicity of Androgen Deprivation Therapy. CurrCardiol Rep. 2021 Jul 3;23(8):109. doi: 10.1007/s11886-021-01561-9. PMID: 34216282; PMCID: PMC8254069.
- Morgans AK, Shore N, Cope D, McNatty A, Moslehi J, Gomella L, Sartor O. Androgen receptor inhibitor treatments: Cardiovascular adverse events and comorbidity considerations in patients with non-metastatic prostate cancer. Urol Oncol. 2021 Jan;39(1):52-62. doi: 10.1016/j.urolonc.2020.08.003. Epub 2020 Sep 18. PMID: 32958445.

24. Which of the following cancer drugs is associated with arterial thrombosis?

    A. Arsenic trioxide
    B. Bleomycin
    C. Ifosfamide
    D. Pazopanib

    Pazopanib is an oral kinase inhibitor targeting vascular endothelial growth factor receptor (VEGFR), platelet-derived growth factor receptor (PDGFR), and c-Kit. It is currently approved in the United States for the treatment of advanced renal cell carcinoma and advanced soft tissue sarcoma who have received prior chemotherapy. Pazopanib is associated with a myriad of adverse effects, and it can particularly affect the cardiovascular system. In VEG105192 trial, the most common adverse effects were grade 1 and 2 and included diarrhea (52%), hypertension (40%), hair color changes (38%), nausea (26%), anorexia (22%), and vomiting (21%). The most common grade 3 and 4 adverse effects were hypertension (4%) and diarrhea (4%). Arterial thromboembolic events occurred in 3% of pazopanib-treated patients: myocardial infarction/ischemia (2%), cerebrovascular accident (<1%), and transient ischemia attack (<1%). The incidence of hemorrhagic events (all grades) in the pazopanib group was 13% compared with 5% in the placebo arm.

U.S. Food and Drug Administration Prescribing Information – Votrient (pazopanib)	
Cardiovascular Main Warnings	**Non-Cardiovascular Main Warnings**
■ Arterial thromboembolic events ■ Venous thromboembolic events ■ Hypertension ■ QT prolongation and torsades de pointes ■ Cardiac dysfunction ■ Hemorrhagic events	■ Hepatic toxicity ■ Gastrointestinal perforation and fistula ■ Thrombotic microangiopathy ■ Interstitial lung disease/ pneumonitis ■ Risk of impaired wound healing ■ Posterior reversible encephalopathy syndrome ■ Proteinuria

Reference(s):

- Novartis Pharmaceuticals Corporation. Votrient (pazopanib) [package insert]. U.S. Food and Drug Administration website. https://www.accessdata.fda.gov/drugsatfda_docs/label/2012/022465s-010S-012lbl.pdf. Revised April 2012. Accessed September 1, 2022.
- Sternberg CN, Davis ID, Mardiak J, Szczylik C, Lee E, Wagstaff J, Barrios CH, Salman P, Gladkov OA, Kavina A, Zarbá JJ, Chen M, McCann L, Pandite L, Roychowdhury DF, Hawkins RE. Pazopanib in locally advanced or metastatic renal cell carcinoma: results of a randomized phase III trial. J Clin Oncol. 2010 Feb 20;28(6):1061-8. doi: 10.1200/JCO.2009.23.9764. Epub 2010 Jan 25. PMID: 20100962.

25. An 83-year-old female with myelodysplastic syndrome who receives frequent blood transfusions presents with worsening dyspnea on exertion. Vital signs showed a pulse of 105 beats per minute, blood pressure of 110/80 mmHg, respiratory rate 18 breaths per minute, and oxygen saturation 98% on 2 liters per minute of supplemental oxygen via nasal cannula. Physical exam demonstrated an elevated jugular venous pressure and bilateral fine crackles with decreased breath sounds. Her N-terminal pro-brain natriuretic peptide (NT-proBNP), ferritin, and transferrin saturation are elevated. Which of the following tests will help the most in establishing the etiology of her presentation?

    A. Cardiac magnetic resonance imaging (MRI)
    B. Echocardiogram with strain imaging
    C. FDG/PET scan
    D. Pyrophosphate scan

    Cardiac dysfunction resulting in heart failure is the most common cause of death in ß-thalassemia major and results from myocardial iron overload. The latter can be seen in other conditions including iron transfusion overload. According to a consensus statement from the American Heart Association regarding the assessment of cardiovascular function and treatment in ß-thalassemia major, the estimation of cardiac iron by cardiac T2* magnetic resonance is key in the diagnosis of prognosis of this condition. Serum ferritin and liver iron concentration are not considered to be adequate surrogates for myocardial iron measurement. A shortening of cardiac T2* to less than 20 milliseconds is associated with an increased likelihood of decreased left ventricular ejection fraction (LVEF), with values of 4 milliseconds associated with a 70% chance of decreased LVEF.

Reference(s):

- Hoffbrand AV, Taher A, Cappellini MD. How I treat transfusional iron overload. Blood. 2012 Nov 1;120(18):3657-69. doi: 10.1182/blood-2012-05-370098. Epub 2012 Aug 23. PMID: 22919029.
- Kwiatkowski JL. Real-world use of iron chelators. Hematology Am Soc Hematol Educ Program. 2011;2011:451-8. doi: 10.1182/asheducation-2011.1.451. PMID: 22160073.

- Meloni A, Martini N, Positano V, De Luca A, Pistoia L, Sbragi S, Spasiano A, Casini T, Bitti PP, Allò M, Sanna PMG, De Caterina R, Sinagra G, Pepe A. Myocardial iron overload by cardiovascular magnetic resonance native segmental T1 mapping: a sensitive approach that correlates with cardiac complications. J Cardiovasc MagnReson. 2021 Jun 14;23(1):70. doi: 10.1186/s12968-021-00765-w. PMID: 34120634; PMCID: PMC8201743.
- Pennell DJ, Udelson JE, Arai AE, Bozkurt B, Cohen AR, Galanello R, Hoffman TM, Kiernan MS, Lerakis S, Piga A, Porter JB, Walker JM, Wood J; American Heart Association Committee on Heart Failure and Transplantation of the Council on Clinical Cardiology and Council on Cardiovascular Radiology and Imaging. Cardiovascular function and treatment in β-thalassemia major: a consensus statement from the American Heart Association. Circulation. 2013 Jul 16;128(3):281-308. doi: 10.1161/CIR.0b013e31829b2be6. Epub 2013 Jun 17. Erratum in: Circulation. 2013 Sep 24;128(13):e203. PMID: 23775258.
- Westwood MA, Anderson LJ, Maceira AM, Shah FT, Prescott E, Porter JB, Wonke B, Walker JM, Pennell DJ. Normalized left ventricular volumes and function in thalassemia major patients with normal myocardial iron. J MagnReson Imaging. 2007 Jun;25(6):1147-51. doi: 10.1002/jmri.20915. PMID: 17520718.

26. A 73-year-old female with history of sinus node dysfunction is diagnosed with invasive ductal carcinoma of the left breast. Adjuvant radiation therapy is recommended. She has a left-sided dual chamber pacemaker and her right ventricular pacing burden is 60%. Which of the following is most associated with radiation-induced device malfunction?

    A. Anatomical location of the tumor (below diaphragm versus above diaphragm)

    B. Cumulative tumor dose

    C. Fraction of radiation therapy courses

    D. High beam energy (≥15 megavolt [MV])

    There are two types of CIED malfunctions: errors in software and in hardware. Software errors refer to changes in the backup settings, oversensing that occurs temporarily only during irradiation, and inappropriate ICD operation. Hardware errors refer to permanent damage to the device requiring replacement. Radiation energies that lead to neutron contamination are the most likely to damage devices. These include photon energy of >10 MV, electron energy >20 MeV, and proton therapy. Since CIED malfunction is due to neutron contamination and neutrons can penetrate significant distances, device relocation is not necessarily protective.

Reference(s):

- Fradley MG, Lefebvre B, Carver J, Cheung JW, Feigenberg SJ, Lampert R, Liu J, Rajagopalan B, Lenihan DJ. How to Manage Patients With Cardiac Implantable Electronic Devices Undergoing Radiation Therapy. JACC CardioOncol. 2021 Sep 21;3(3):447-451. doi: 10.1016/j.jaccao.2021.08.005. PMID: 34604807; PMCID: PMC8463726.
- Toshiki Ohno, ToshinoriSoejima, Yukio Sekiguchi, Takayuki Hashimoto, Izumi Koike, Hiroaki Matsubara, Kazuhiko Nakamura, Kazunori Nitta, Shigeo

Takahashi, Kayoko Tsujino, Masaru Wakatsuki, EisakuYoden, JASTRO/JCS Guidelines for radiotherapy in patients with cardiac implantable electronic devices, *Journal of Radiation Research*, Volume 62, Issue 1, January 2021, Pages 172–184, doi.org/10.1093/jrr/rraa102.

27. Which of the following is the proposed mechanism for ibrutinib-induced atrial fibrillation?

A. Decreased resveratrol production

B. Enhanced potassium channel blockade

C. Inhibition of C-terminal SRC kinase

D. Inhibition of platelet-derived growth factor (PDGF) signaling

A study using murine models showed that ibrutinib-mediated atrial fibrillation is attributable to off-target inhibition of CSK. Cardiac specific CSK knockout mice led to increase atrial fibrillation, left atrial enlargement, fibrosis, and inflammation, similar to the effects of ibrutinib treatment.

Reference(s):

- Xiao L, Salem JE, Clauss S, Hanley A, Bapat A, Hulsmans M, Iwamoto Y, Wojtkiewicz G, Cetinbas M, Schloss MJ, Tedeschi J, Lebrun-Vignes B, Lundby A, Sadreyev RI, Moslehi J, Nahrendorf M, Ellinor PT, Milan DJ. Ibrutinib-Mediated Atrial Fibrillation Attributable to Inhibition of C-Terminal Src Kinase. Circulation. 2020 Dec 22;142(25):2443-2455. doi: 10.1161/CIRCULATIONAHA.120.049210. Epub 2020 Oct 23. PMID: 33092403.

28. Which of the following is considered a clinically acceptable maximum radiation dose to pacemakers and defibrillators?

A. 2 to 5 grays (Gy)

B. 11 to 20 Gy

C. 25 to 30 Gy

D. Less than 1 Gy

The tolerance radiation dose for a cardiac implantable electronic device (CIED) to prevent malfunction has not been clearly defined. Until August 2018, each manufacturer specified device dose limits of ≤5 Gy. The medical physicist should estimate the absorbed dose to the device as part of treatment planning.

Reference(s):

- Fradley MG, Lefebvre B, Carver J, Cheung JW, Feigenberg SJ, Lampert R, Liu J, Rajagopalan B, Lenihan DJ. How to Manage Patients With Cardiac Implantable Electronic Devices Undergoing Radiation Therapy. JACC CardioOncol. 2021 Sep 21;3(3):447-451. doi: 10.1016/j.jaccao.2021.08.005. PMID: 34604807; PMCID: PMC8463726.
- Toshiki Ohno, ToshinoriSoejima, Yukio Sekiguchi, Takayuki Hashimoto, Izumi Koike, Hiroaki Matsubara, Kazuhiko Nakamura, Kazunori Nitta, Shigeo Takahashi, Kayoko Tsujino, Masaru Wakatsuki, EisakuYoden, JASTRO/JCS Guidelines for radiotherapy in patients with cardiac implantable electronic

devices, *Journal of Radiation Research*, Volume 62, Issue 1, January 2021, Pages 172–184, doi.org/10.1093/jrr/rraa102.

29. Which of the following cancer type has the highest points when calculating the Khorana score?

A. Lung
B. Lymphoma
C. Pancreas
D. Prostate

Variables	Risk score
Cancer type	
■ Very high risk (stomach, pancreas)	2
■ High risk (lung, lymphoma, gynecologic, bladder, testicular)	1
Pre-chemotherapy platelet count, ≥350 x 10^9/L	1
Hemoglobin level <10 g/dL or using RBC growth factors	1
Pre-chemotherapy leukocyte count >11 x 10^9/L	1
Body mass index ≥35 kg/m^2	1

Three risk categories were defined based on the score from the risk model: low (score 0), intermediate (1-2), and high (≥3). The model was validated in an independent cohort of patients from the same observational study. In the validation cohort, the rates of symptomatic venous thromboembolism over a median period of follow up of 2.5 months were 0.3% in the low-risk category, 2% in the intermediate-risk category, and 6.7% in the high-risk category.

Reference(s):

- Khorana AA, Kuderer NM, Culakova E, Lyman GH, Francis CW. Development and validation of a predictive model for chemotherapy-associated thrombosis. Blood. 2008 May 15;111(10):4902-7. doi: 10.1182/blood-2007-10-116327. Epub 2008 Jan 23. PMID: 18216292; PMCID: PMC2384124.

30. Which of the following oral anticoagulants have been effective at primary prevention of venous thromboembolism in patients with cancer and a Khorana score of ≥2?

A. Apixaban and dabigatran
B. Apixaban and rivaroxaban
C. Edoxaban and dabigatran
D. Edoxaban and rivaroxaban

The AVERT trial was a randomized, placebo-controlled, double-blind clinical trial comparing apixaban (2.5 mg twice daily) with placebo for thromboprophylaxis in ambulatory patients with cancer who were at intermediate-to-high risk for venous thromboembolism (VTE) based on a Khorana score ≥2, and were starting chemotherapy. The primary efficacy outcome was objectively documented VTE over a follow-up period of 180 days. VTE occurred in 12 of 288 patients (4.2%) in the apixaban group and in 28 of 275 patients (10.2%) in the placebo group (hazard ratio, 0.41; 95% confidence interval [CI], 0.26 to 0.65; $p < 0.001$).

The CASSINI trial was a randomized, double-blind, placebo-controlled, parallel-group, phase 3b trial comparing rivaroxaban (10 mg daily) with placebo for thromboprophylaxis in ambulatory patients with cancer and a Khorana score ≥2. The primary efficacy end point was a composite of objectively confirmed proximal deep vein thrombosis (DVT) in a lower limb, pulmonary embolism, symptomatic DVT in an upper limb or distal DVT in a lower limb, and death from VTE over a follow-up period of 180 days. The primary end point occurred in 25 of 420 patients (6.0%) in the rivaroxaban group and in 37 of 421 (8.8%) in the placebo group (hazard ratio, 0.66; 95% CI, 0.40 to 1.09; $p = 0.1$) in the period up to day 180. However, in the prespecified intervention-period analysis, the primary end point occurred in 11 patients (2.6%) in the rivaroxaban group and in 27 (6.4%) in the placebo group (hazard ratio, 0.4; 95% CI, 0.20 to 0.80).

Edoxaban and dabigatran have not been studied in this setting (thromboprophylaxis in patients with cancer).

Reference(s):

- Carrier M, Abou-Nassar K, Mallick R, Tagalakis V, Shivakumar S, Schattner A, Kuruvilla P, Hill D, Spadafora S, Marquis K, Trinkaus M, Tomiak A, Lee AYY, Gross PL, Lazo-Langner A, El-Maraghi R, Goss G, Le Gal G, Stewart D, Ramsay T, Rodger M, Witham D, Wells PS; AVERT Investigators. Apixaban to Prevent Venous Thromboembolism in Patients with Cancer. N Engl J Med. 2019 Feb 21;380(8):711-719. doi: 10.1056/NEJMoa1814468. Epub 2018 Dec 4. PMID: 30511879.
- Khorana AA, Soff GA, Kakkar AK, Vadhan-Raj S, Riess H, Wun T, Streiff MB, Garcia DA, Liebman HA, Belani CP, O'Reilly EM, Patel JN, Yimer HA, Wildgoose P, Burton P, Vijapurkar U, Kaul S, Eikelboom J, McBane R, Bauer KA, Kuderer NM, Lyman GH; CASSINI Investigators. Rivaroxaban for Thromboprophylaxis in High-Risk Ambulatory Patients with Cancer. N Engl J Med. 2019 Feb 21;380(8):720-728. doi: 10.1056/NEJMoa1814630. PMID: 30786186.

31. In which of the following cases is prophylaxis for venous thromboembolism recommended by the American Society of Clinical Oncology?

    A. Breast cancer treatment with exemestane

    B. Melanoma treatment with nivolumab and ipilimumab

    C. Multiple myeloma treatment with lenalidomide

    D. Non-small cell lung cancer treatment with bevacizumab

The American Society of Hematology 2021 guidelines for management of venous thromboembolism (VTE) in patients with cancer suggests using low-dose acetylsalicylic acid (ASA) or fixed low-dose vitamin K antagonist (VKA) or low-molecular weight heparin (LMWH) in patients with multiple myeloma receiving lenalidomide, thalidomide, or pomalidomide-based regimens. The expert panel indicated that when cost and feasibility are less of a concern, LMWH may be the better choice, especially in patients considered at higher risk for VTE. They acknowledged that subcutaneous administration of LMWH over a long period of time may not be acceptable to some patients. They further recognized an increased risk for bleeding in patients on ASA who are also receiving steroids. The panel indicated that there is low-certainty evidence of a "net health benefit from low-dose ASA over fixed-dose VKA thromboprophylaxis and concluded that the balance of effects does not favor either." Regarding ASA over LMWH thromboprophylaxis, the panel concluded that the balance of effects probably favors LMWH.

Reference(s):

- Lyman GH, Carrier M, Ay C, Di Nisio M, Hicks LK, Khorana AA, Leavitt AD, Lee AYY, Macbeth F, Morgan RL, Noble S, Sexton EA, Stenehjem D, Wiercioch W, Kahale LA, Alonso-Coello P. American Society of Hematology 2021 guidelines for management of venous thromboembolism: prevention and treatment in patients with cancer. Blood Adv. 2021 Feb 23;5(4):927-974. doi: 10.1182/bloodadvances.2020003442. Erratum in: Blood Adv. 2021 Apr 13;5(7):1953. PMID: 33570602; PMCID: PMC7903232.

32. A 64-year-old male with angioimmunoblastic T-cell lymphoma presents with worsening shortness of breath. He was treated with CHOP (cyclophosphamide, doxorubicin, vincristine, and prednisone), and 2 months later with BEAM (carmustine, etoposide, cytarabine, and melphalan) conditioning and autologous stem cell transplantation. A transthoracic echocardiogram was unremarkable. A chest CT scan 3 weeks after the transplant showed bilateral upper lobe ground-glass opacities and scattered pulmonary nodules. Vital signs revealed a pulse of 95 beats per minute, blood pressure of 110/60 mmHg, afebrile, and oxygen saturation of 93% on room air. Which of the following could explain the patient's clinical presentation?

    A. Carmustine

    B. Cyclophosphamide

    C. Doxorubicin

    D. Vincristine

    In a single-center study involving 222 consecutive patients receiving high-dose chemotherapy and autologous stem cell transplantation using cyclophosphamide, carmustine (BCNU), and VP-16, the incidence of pneumonitis was 22%, with 19% receiving systemic steroid treatment and 8% requiring inpatient hospitalization. The authors identified 3 variables that were independently associated with pneumonitis: prior mediastinal radiation, total BCNU dose above 1000 mg, and age less than 54 years.

    Melphalan has also been reported to rarely cause interstitial pneumonitis and fibrosis. This is based on multiple case reports.

Reference(s):

- Akasheh MS, Freytes CO, Vesole DH. Melphalan-associated pulmonary toxicity following high-dose therapy with autologous hematopoietic stem cell transplantation. Bone Marrow Transplant. 2000 Nov;26(10):1107-9. doi: 10.1038/sj.bmt.1702664. PMID: 11108311.

- Lane AA, Armand P, Feng Y, Neuberg DS, Abramson JS, Brown JR, Fisher DC, LaCasce AS, Jacobsen ED, McAfee SL, Spitzer TR, Freedman AS, Chen YB. Risk factors for development of pneumonitis after high-dose chemotherapy with cyclophosphamide, BCNU and etoposide followed by autologous stem cell transplant. Leuk Lymphoma. 2012 Jun;53(6):1130-6. doi: 10.3109/10428194.2011.645208. Epub 2012 Jan 3. PMID: 22132836; PMCID: PMC3376378.

33. Compared with dalteparin (low molecular weight heparin), which of the following statements is true regarding the use of an oral factor Xa inhibitor (rivaroxaban) in patients with cancer and venous thromboembolism (VTE)?

    A. Rivaroxaban is associated with a higher 6-month cumulative rate of VTE recurrence and non-major bleeding.
    B. Rivaroxaban is associated with a higher 6-month cumulative rate of VTE recurrence, but a lower rate of non-major bleeding.
    C. Rivaroxaban is associated with a lower 6-month cumulative rate of VTE recurrence, but a higher rate of non-major bleeding.
    D. Rivaroxaban is associated with lower 6-month cumulative rate of VTE recurrence and non-major bleeding.

The SELECT-D trial was a multicenter, randomized, open-label, pilot trial in the United Kingdom that included 203 patients with active cancer who had symptomatic pulmonary embolism (PE), incidental PE, or symptomatic lower extremity deep vein thrombosis (DVT). Patients were randomized to dalteparin or rivaroxaban (15 mg twice daily for 3 weeks, then 20 mg once daily for a total of 6 months). The primary outcome was venous thromboembolism (VTE) recurrence over 6 months. Safety end points included major bleeding and clinically relevant nonmajor bleeding (CRNMB). The 6-month cumulative VTE recurrence rate was 11% (95% confidence interval [CI], 7% to 16%) with dalteparin and 4% (95% CI, 2% to 9%) with rivaroxaban (hazard ratio [HR], 0.43; 95% CI, 0.19 to 0.99). The 6-month cumulative rate of major bleeding was 4% (95% CI, 2% to 8%) for dalteparin and 6% (95% CI, 3% to 11%) for rivaroxaban (HR, 1.83; 95% CI, 0.68 to 4.96). Rates of CRNMB were 4% (95% CI, 2% to 9%) for dalteparin and 13% (95% CI, 9% to 19%) for rivaroxaban (HR, 3.76; 95% CI, 1.63 to 8.69). Rivaroxaban was shown to be associated with a relatively low VTE recurrence but higher CRNMB compared with dalteparin.

Reference(s):

- Young AM, Marshall A, Thirlwall J, Chapman O, Lokare A, Hill C, Hale D, Dunn JA, Lyman GH, Hutchinson C, MacCallum P, Kakkar A, Hobbs FDR, Petrou S, Dale J, Poole CJ, Maraveyas A, Levine M. Comparison of an Oral Factor Xa Inhibitor With Low Molecular Weight Heparin in Patients With Cancer With Venous Thromboembolism: Results of a Randomized Trial (SELECT-D). J Clin Oncol. 2018 Jul 10;36(20):2017-2023. doi: 10.1200/JCO.2018.78.8034. Epub 2018 May 10. PMID: 29746227.

34. According to the American College of Cardiology and American Heart Association, in what stage of heart failure are asymptomatic patients with no structural heart disease after receiving cardiotoxic treatment classified?

    A. Stage A
    B. Stage B
    C. Stage C
    D. Stage D

American College of Cardiology and American Heart Association Stages of Heart Failure

Stages	Description and Criteria
Stage A At risk for heart failure	■ At risk for HF but without symptoms, structural heart disease, or abnormal cardiac biomarkers ■ Examples: hypertension, atherosclerotic cardiovascular disease, diabetes, metabolic syndrome and obesity, exposure to cardiotoxic agents (e.g., chemotherapy such as anthracyclines), genetic variant for cardiomyopathy, or positive family history of cardiomyopathy
Stage B Pre-heart failure	■ No symptoms or signs of HF, but with evidence of 1 of the following: ✓ Structural heart disease • Reduced left or right ventricular systolic function (reduced ejection fraction, reduced strain) • Ventricular hypertrophy • Chamber enlargement • Wall motion abnormalities • Valvular heart disease ✓ Evidence for increased filling pressures • By invasive hemodynamic measurements • By noninvasive imaging suggesting elevated filling pressures (e.g., Doppler echocardiography) ✓ Risk factors and increased levels of B-type natriuretic peptide or persistently elevated cardiac troponin (in the absence of other diagnoses such as acute coronary syndrome, chronic kidney disease, pulmonary embolus, or myopericarditis)
Stage C Symptomatic heart failure	■ Structural heart disease with current or previous symptoms of HF

Stages	Description and Criteria
Stage D Advanced heart failure	■ Severe HF symptoms impairing activities of daily living and recurrent hospitalizations despite appropriate guideline-directed medical therapy ■ Patients being considered for advanced therapies such as heart transplantation and/or left ventricular assist device

Reference(s):

- Heidenreich PA, Bozkurt B, Aguilar D, Allen LA, Byun JJ, Colvin MM, Deswal A, Drazner MH, Dunlay SM, Evers LR, Fang JC, Fedson SE, Fonarow GC, Hayek SS, Hernandez AF, Khazanie P, Kittleson MM, Lee CS, Link MS, Milano CA, Nnacheta LC, Sandhu AT, Stevenson LW, Vardeny O, Vest AR, Yancy CW. 2022 AHA/ACC/HFSA Guideline for the Management of Heart Failure: A Report of the American College of Cardiology/American Heart Association Joint Committee on Clinical Practice Guidelines. Circulation. 2022 May 3;145(18):e895-e1032. doi: 10.1161/CIR.0000000000001063. Epub 2022 Apr 1. Erratum in: Circulation. 2022 May 3;145(18):e1033. Erratum in: Circulation. 2022 Sep 27;146(13):e185. PMID: 35363499.

35. Which of the following iron chelators may be useful to prevent cardiac dysfunction in patients receiving doxorubicin?

A. Deferasirox

B. Deferiprone

C. Deferoxamine

D. Dexrazoxane

In a phase II single-arm non-inferiority trial consisting of 33 patients with metastatic or unresectable soft tissue sarcoma (STS) receiving doxorubicin (cycles of 75 mg/m^2 every 21 days) with or without olaratumab, dexrazoxane (administered in a 10:1 ratio to doxorubicin (750 mg/m^2) was started with cycle 1 and continued through the duration of the study. Over a median of 16.1 months of follow-up (interquartile range [IQR], 5.7-25 months), progression-free survival (PFS) was a median of 8.4 months (IQR, 4-11.2 months). At the time of interim analysis, 6 patients had not yet progressed. There were 13 deaths (12 due to cancer progression and 1 due to myocarditis in a patient who received checkpoint inhibitor therapy after progressing on study protocol). There were no deaths attributed to doxorubicin. Patients received a median of 6 cycles (450 mg/m^2; IQR, 300-750 mg/m^2) of doxorubicin prior to interim analysis. The number of cycles ranged from 1 to 38. Five patients received over 1,000 mg/m^2 of doxorubicin, with 2 patients receiving over 2,000 mg/m^2 to a maximum of 2,850 mg/m^2. Of these 5 patients, only 1 was taken off study for cardiotoxicity and 4 were removed due to disease progression. Among the entire study cohort, there was no difference between LVEF measured at baseline, at the end of the study treatment, and at the end of the follow-up period. Dexrazoxane did not reduce PFS.

Reference(s):

- Van Tine BA, Hirbe AC, Oppelt P, Frith AE, Rathore R, Mitchell JD, Wan F, Berry S, Landeau M, Heberton GA, Gorcsan J 3rd, Huntjens PR, Soyama Y, Vader JM, Alvarez-Cardona JA, Zhang KW, Lenihan DJ, Krone RJ. Interim Analysis of the Phase II Study: Noninferiority Study of Doxorubicin with Upfront Dexrazoxane plus Olaratumab for Advanced or Metastatic Soft-Tissue Sarcoma. Clin Cancer Res. 2021 Jul 15;27(14):3854-3860. doi: 10.1158/1078-0432.CCR-20-4621. Epub 2021 Mar 25. PMID: 33766818; PMCID: PMC8282681.

36. Compared to photon therapy, which of the following is true regarding the use of proton therapy in patients with cancer?

    A. Proton therapy has been shown to improve overall survival in patients with locally advanced cancer.

    B. Proton therapy is associated with a reduction in adverse effects.

    C. Proton therapy results in a higher risk of decline in performance status.

    D. Proton therapy results in a similar amount of radiation exposure.

    In a retrospective, nonrandomized comparative effectiveness study including 1,483 adult patients with non-metastatic, locally advanced cancer treated with concurrent chemoradiotherapy with curative intent, 391 patients received proton therapy and 1,092 photon therapy. Proton chemoradiotherapy was associated with significantly reduced acute adverse events with similar disease-free and overall survival.

Reference(s):

- Baumann BC, Mitra N, Harton JG, Xiao Y, Wojcieszynski AP, Gabriel PE, Zhong H, Geng H, Doucette A, Wei J, O'Dwyer PJ, Bekelman JE, Metz JM. Comparative Effectiveness of Proton vs Photon Therapy as Part of Concurrent Chemoradiotherapy for Locally Advanced Cancer. JAMA Oncol. 2020 Feb 1;6(2):237-246. doi: 10.1001/jamaoncol.2019.4889. PMID: 31876914; PMCID: PMC6990870.

37. Which of the following statements is correct regarding radiation-induced heart disease?

    A. Right-sided cardiac valves are more often involved versus left-sided.

    B. The extent of aorto-mitral curtain thickening and/or calcification is associated with surgical mortality.

    C. The left bundle branch is more susceptible to the effects of radiation than the right bundle branch.

    D. Valvular heart disease usually manifests earlier than coronary artery disease.

    Mediastinal or thoracic radiation leads to radiation-associated cardiac disease (RACD). This is associated with multiple complications including conduction rhythm disturbances, valvular heart disease, pericardial and myocardial disease, and coronary artery disease, among others. One-hundred and seventy-three patients with RACD (75% women, 63 ± 14 years, 53% with breast cancer, 27% with Hodgkin lymphoma, mean time from radiation 18 ±12 years) underwent cardiothoracic surgery (26% were redo) between 2000 and 2003. The majority of the patients had valve disease. In addition to other factors, the aorto-mitral curtain (AMC) thickness independently predicted mortality, especially when at least 0.6 cm thick.

Reference(s):

- Desai MY, Wu W, Masri A, Popovic ZB, Agarwal S, Smedira NG, Lytle BW, Griffin BP. Increased aorto-mitral curtain thickness independently predicts mortality in patients with radiation-associated cardiac disease undergoing cardiac surgery. Ann Thorac Surg. 2014 Apr;97(4):1348-55. doi: 10.1016/j.athoracsur.2013.12.029. Epub 2014 Feb 22. PMID: 24565403.

38. Which of the following genetic mutations associated with the development of a dilated cardiomyopathy has also been found to carry a higher risk for the development of anthracycline-induced cardiotoxicity?

    A. Lamin A/C (LMNA)

    B. Sodium channel SCN5A

    C. Titin-truncating variants

    D. TNNT2

    In a study consisting of patients with cancer therapy-induced cardiomyopathy (CCM), there was an increased prevalence of dilated cardiomyopathy-associated gene variants, particularly titin-truncating variants (TTNtvs). TTNtvs were identified in 16 of 213 CCM cases (7.5%). Ninety percent of the 213 patients with CCM had been treated with anthracyclines. Adult patients who had CCM with TTNtvs experienced more heart failure and atrial fibrillation than those without.

Reference(s):

- Garcia-Pavia P, Kim Y, Restrepo-Cordoba MA, Lunde IG, Wakimoto H, Smith AM, Toepfer CN, Getz K, Gorham J, Patel P, Ito K, Willcox JA, Arany Z, Li J, Owens AT, Govind R, Nuñez B, Mazaika E, Bayes-Genis A, Walsh R, Finkelman B, Lupon J, Whiffin N, Serrano I, Midwinter W, Wilk A, Bardaji A, Ingold N, Buchan R, Tayal U, Pascual-Figal DA, de Marvao A, Ahmad M, Garcia-Pinilla JM, Pantazis A, Dominguez F, John Baksi A, O'Regan DP, Rosen SD, Prasad SK, Lara-Pezzi E, Provencio M, Lyon AR, Alonso-Pulpon L, Cook SA, DePalma SR, Barton PJR, Aplenc R, Seidman JG, Ky B, Ware JS, Seidman CE. Genetic Variants Associated With Cancer Therapy-Induced Cardiomyopathy. Circulation. 2019 Jul 2;140(1):31-41. doi: 10.1161/CIRCULATIONAHA.118.037934. Epub 2019 Apr 16. PMID: 30987448; PMCID: PMC6613726.

39. Which of the following statements is most accurate regarding the outcome of patients with severe aortic stenosis after chest radiation therapy?

    A. Post-procedural atrial fibrillation is more common in transcatheter aortic valve replacement (TAVR) than in surgical aortic valve replacement (SAVR).

    B. SAVR is associated with a shorter hospital stay when compared to TAVR.

    C. SAVR is associated with a lower adjusted 1-year all-cause mortality when compared to TAVR in this patient population.

    D. TAVR is associated with a lower adjusted 30-day all-cause mortality.

Guha and colleagues investigated the effect modification of cancer on the relative use rate, outcomes, and dispositions associated with propensity-matched cohort transcatheter aortic valve replacement (TAVR) versus surgical aortic valve replacement (SAVR). They queried the US-based National Inpatient Sample for patients aged ≥50 years with a primary diagnosis of aortic stenosis. Among patients with cancer, TAVR was associated with lower odds of acute kidney injury and major bleeding, with no differences in in-hospital mortality and stroke compared with SAVR. TAVR was also associated with higher odds of home discharge compared with SAVR among patients with cancer.

Another study by Lind and colleagues determined the impact of cancer on peri-procedural complications and survival in a total of 1,088 patients (839 controls, 196 with stable cancer, and 53 with active cancer). No significant differences were observed regarding peri-procedural complications. Patients with active cancer had similar 30-day survival compared with controls and stable cancer patients, but a reduced 10-year survival.

A retrospective analysis comparing 30-day outcomes of TAVR versus SAVR in patients with severe aortic stenosis and a prior history of mediastinal radiation showed that TAVR was associated with a significantly reduced 30-day mortality (odds ratio 0.6, 0.4-0.91), postoperative atrial fibrillation, pneumonia, pleural effusion, renal failure, and bleeding. However, stroke/transient ischemic attack and pacemaker implantation were higher with TAVR.

Reference(s):

- Guha A, Dey AK, Arora S, Cavender MA, Vavalle JP, Sabik JF III,, Jimenez E, Jneid H, Addison D. Contemporary Trends and Outcomes of Percutaneous and Surgical Aortic Valve Replacement in Patients With Cancer. J Am Heart Assoc. 2020 Jan 21;9(2):e014248. doi: 10.1161/JAHA.119.014248. Epub 2020 Jan 21. PMID: 31960751; PMCID: PMC7033818.
- Lind A, Totzeck M, Mahabadi AA, Jánosi RA, El Gabry M, Ruhparwar A, Mrotzek SM, Hinrichs L, Akdeniz M, Rassaf T, Mincu RI. Impact of Cancer in Patients Undergoing Transcatheter Aortic Valve Replacement: A Single-Center Study. JACC CardioOncol. 2020 Dec 15;2(5):735-743. doi: 10.1016/j.jaccao.2020.11.008. PMID: 34396288; PMCID: PMC8352296.
- Nauffal V, Bay C, Shah PB, Sobieszczyk PS, Kaneko T, O'Gara P, Nohria A. Short-Term Outcomes of Transcatheter Versus Isolated Surgical Aortic Valve Replacement for Mediastinal Radiation-Associated Severe Aortic Stenosis. Circ Cardiovasc Interv. 2021 Feb;14(2):e010009. doi: 10.1161/CIRCINTERVENTIONS.120.010009. Epub 2021 Feb 5. PMID: 33541102.

40. A 60-year-old male presents to the Cardio-Oncology Clinic for evaluation of an elevated resting heart rate. The patient has history of Hodgkin's lymphoma treated with thoracic radiation therapy and anthracycline-containing chemotherapy 20 years ago. Which of the following statements is correct regarding previous treatment with thoracic radiation and the development of autonomic dysfunction?

A. Abnormal heart rate recovery predicts increased all-cause mortality in survivors treated with thoracic radiation therapy.
B. Autonomic dysfunction is associated with the presence of cardiovascular risk factors.
C. Autonomic dysfunction is characterized by increased parasympathetic and attenuated sympathetic activity.
D. Prevalence of autonomic dysfunction is independent of time from thoracic radiation therapy.

In a retrospective study evaluating the prevalence of autonomic dysfunction and its implications on exercise capacity and mortality in long-term survivors of Hodgkin lymphoma, thoracic radiotherapy was associated with autonomic dysfunction and consequently, impaired exercise tolerance and abnormal heart rate recovery. The latter was shown to predict increased all-cause mortality in patients treated with radiotherapy. Prevalence of autonomic dysfunction increased with radiation dose and time from treatment.

Reference(s):

- Groarke JD, Tanguturi VK, Hainer J, Klein J, Moslehi JJ, Ng A, Forman DE, Di Carli MF, Nohria A. Abnormal exercise response in long-term survivors of hodgkin lymphoma treated with thoracic irradiation: evidence of cardiac autonomic dysfunction and impact on outcomes. J Am Coll Cardiol. 2015 Feb 17;65(6):573-83. doi: 10.1016/j.jacc.2014.11.035. PMID: 25677317.

41. Which of the following interventions is associated with a significant reduction in stroke in patients treated with radiation therapy to the head, neck, and thorax?

A. Atorvastatin
B. Fish oil
C. Lisinopril
D. Metoprolol

Among patients with thorax and head or neck cancer having undergone radiotherapy between 2000 and 2011, statin use post radiotherapy was associated with a significant reduction in stroke (hazard ratio = 0.68; 95% confidence interval, 0.48-0.98; p = 0.0368).

Reference(s):

- Boulet J, Peña J, Hulten EA, Neilan TG, Dragomir A, Freeman C, Lambert C, Hijal T, Nadeau L, Brophy JM, Mousavi N. Statin Use and Risk of Vascular Events Among Cancer Patients After Radiotherapy to the Thorax, Head, and Neck. J Am Heart Assoc. 2019 Jul 2;8(13):e005996. doi: 10.1161/JAHA.117.005996. Epub 2019 Jun 19. PMID: 31213106; PMCID: PMC6662340.

42. A 45-year-old female with hormone-receptor-positive breast cancer is started on adjuvant endocrine therapy. Which of the following is most accurate regarding the risk of venous thromboembolism (VTE) among breast cancer survivors treated with adjuvant endocrine therapy?

A. Both tamoxifen and aromatase inhibitors have a similar risk of VTE.

B. Tamoxifen is associated with a higher risk of VTE compared to an aromatase inhibitor.

C. Aromatase inhibitors are associated with a higher VTE risk than tamoxifen.

D. There is no increased risk of VTE.

In a prospective cohort study of 12,904 postmenopausal women who were diagnosed with a first primary hormone-receptor-positive breast cancer and free from previous cardiovascular disease or VTE from 1991 to 2010, aromatase inhibitor use was associated with at least 41% lower VTE risk compared to tamoxifen use during a median of 5.4 years follow-up (adjusted hazard ratio 0.59; 95% confidence interval, 0.43-0.81). The authors also found an even lower risk of VTE in women who received chemotherapy and in women with stage I-III disease.

Reference(s):

- Xu X, Chlebowski RT, Shi J, Barac A, Haque R. Aromatase inhibitor and tamoxifen use and the risk of venous thromboembolism in breast cancer survivors. Breast Cancer Res Treat. 2019 Apr;174(3):785-794. doi: 10.1007/s10549-018-05086-8. Epub 2019 Jan 18. PMID: 30659431.

43. Among patients with prostate cancer and high baseline cardiovascular (CV) risk, prolonged exposure (more than 6 months) to androgen deprivation therapy (ADT) has been associated with:

A. Good cardiorespiratory fitness (CRF), but reduced CV mortality

B. Good CRF and paradoxical increased CV mortality

C. Reduced CRF and increased CV mortality

D. Reduced CRF and no significant effect on CV mortality

Gong and colleagues designed a retrospective cohort study to compare CRF and CV mortality among patients with prostate cancer with and without ADT exposure and to explore how duration of ADT exposure influences CRT and CV mortality. Prostate cancer risk classification was based on Gleason score; CRT was categorized by metabolic equivalents; and ADT exposure was defined as short term ($\leq$6 months) versus prolonged (>6 months). A total of 616 patients underwent an exercise treadmill stress test at a median of 4.8 years (interquartile range: 2.0 – 7.9 years) after their diagnosis of prostate cancer. The authors found that among patients with prostate cancer and high baseline cardiovascular risk (defined as having $\geq$2 risk factors), prolonged ADT exposure was associated with reduced CRF (odds ratio, 2.71; 95% confidence interval, 1.31 – 5.61; $p = 0.007$) and increased CV mortality (hazard ratio, 3.87; 95% confidence interval 1.15 – 12.96; $p = 0.028$).

Reference(s):

- Gong J, Payne D, Caron J, Bay CP, McGregor BA, Hainer J, Partridge AH, Neilan TG, Di Carli M, Nohria A, Groarke JD. Reduced Cardiorespiratory Fitness and Increased Cardiovascular Mortality After Prolonged Androgen Deprivation Therapy for Prostate Cancer. JACC CardioOncol. 2020 Nov 17;2(4):553-563. doi: 10.1016/j.jaccao.2020.08.011. PMID: 34396266; PMCID: PMC8352085.

44. What is the recommended duration of anticoagulation for the treatment of cancer-associated venous thromboembolic disease?

A. At least 1 month

B. At least 3 months

C. At least 6 months

D. At least 12 months

According to the American Society of Hematology (ASH) 2021 guidelines for management of venous thromboembolism (VTE) in patients with cancer, long-term anticoagulation (>6 months) for secondary VTE prophylaxis should be considered in patients with active cancer in the absence of contraindications to anticoagulation. The ASH guideline panel suggests using a direct oral anticoagulant (e.g., apixaban, rivaroxaban) or low-molecular-weight heparin (LMWH). Long-term anticoagulation can be discontinued when patients are no longer considered at high risk for recurrent VTEs or if patients are entering the last weeks of life. Other aspects to consider include type and stage of cancer, overall prognosis, risk of bleeding, costs and patients' preferences, and potential drug-drug interactions. Long-term anticoagulation (>6 months) or indefinite anticoagulation have not been shown to impact mortality, but may decrease recurrent VTEs. No specific trial has addressed this question, and the panel identified this as an important knowledge gap.

Reference(s):

- Lyman GH, Carrier M, Ay C, Di Nisio M, Hicks LK, Khorana AA, Leavitt AD, Lee AYY, Macbeth F, Morgan RL, Noble S, Sexton EA, Stenehjem D, Wiercioch W, Kahale LA, Alonso-Coello P. American Society of Hematology 2021 guidelines for management of venous thromboembolism: prevention and treatment in patients with cancer. Blood Adv. 2021 Feb 23;5(4):927-974. doi: 10.1182/bloodadvances.2020003442. Erratum in: Blood Adv. 2021 Apr 13;5(7):1953. PMID: 33570602; PMCID: PMC7903232.

45. There are several proposed mechanisms responsible for the significant hypertensive response seen with vascular endothelial growth factor (VEGF) inhibitors. Which of the following is the most accurate explanation for this effect?

A. A functional increase in nitric oxide production

B. A reduction in endothelin-1 activity

C. A substantial increase in vascular resistance and left ventricular afterload

D. An increase in capillary density as that seen in anatomic rarefaction

In a multicenter, prospective study, 84 patients with metastatic renal cell carcinoma underwent echocardiography, arterial tonometry, and B-type natriuretic peptide (BNP) measures at baseline and at 3.5, 15, and 33 weeks after sunitinib initiation. After 3.5 weeks of sunitinib, mean systolic and diastolic blood pressure increased by 9.5 mmHg (95% confidence interval [CI], 2.0 – 17.1; $p = 0.02$) and 7.2 mmHg (95% CI, 4.3 – 10.0; $p < 0.001$), respectively. Large artery stiffness, resistive load, and pulsatile load also increased. Baseline vascular function parameters were associated with worsening diastolic function and filling pressures over time (but not systolic function).

Reference(s):

- Catino AB, Hubbard RA, Chirinos JA, Townsend R, Keefe S, Haas NB, Puzanov I, Fang JC, Agarwal N, Hyman D, Smith AM, Gordon M, Plappert T, Englefield V, Narayan V, Ewer S, ElAmm C, Lenihan D, Ky B. Longitudinal Assessment of Vascular Function With Sunitinib in Patients With Metastatic Renal Cell Carcinoma. Circ Heart Fail. 2018 Mar;11(3):e004408. doi: 10.1161/CIRCHEARTFAILURE.117.004408. PMID: 29664405; PMCID: PMC6360089.

46. A 64-year-old female with metastatic breast cancer presents with worsening shortness of breath. A chest X-ray shows an enlarged cardiac silhouette. A transthoracic echocardiogram shows a large, circumferential pericardial effusion with indeterminate hemodynamic measurements for tamponade. Physical examination shows an elevated jugular venous pressure. What is the best next step?

    A. Obtain a cardiac magnetic resonance imaging (MRI) with gadolinium contrast

    B. Perform a pericardiocentesis and send sample for cytology

    C. Perform a right and left heart catheterization

    D. Repeat a transthoracic echocardiogram in 6 weeks

    In a study conducted at MD Anderson Cancer Center including 1,645 patients with cancer, 212 (13%) underwent percutaneous pericardiocentesis for a pericardial effusion. The procedure was successful in 99% of the cases, and there were no procedure-related deaths. Four patients had major procedure-related bleeding that was independent of their platelet count (<50,000/μL or ≥50,000/μL). patients with extended catheter drainage for 3 to 5 days had the lowest recurrence rate (10%). Older age (>65 years), lung cancer, platelet count <20,000/μL, and malignant pericardial fluid were independently associated with poor prognosis.

    The patient presented in this clinical vignette would benefit from a pericardiocentesis for symptomatic relief and diagnostic and prognostic utility. Breast cancer is associated with malignant pericardial effusions.

Reference(s):

- Besnard A, Raoux F, Khelil N, Monin JL, Saal JP, Veugeois A, Zannis K, Debauchez M, Caussin C, Amabile N. Current Management of Symptomatic Pericardial Effusions in Cancer Patients. JACC CardioOncol. 2019 Jul 18;1(1):137-140. doi: 10.1016/j.jaccao.2019.07.001. PMID: 34396173; PMCID: PMC8352300.
- El Haddad D, Iliescu C, Yusuf SW, William WN Jr, Khair TH, Song J, Mouhayar EN. Outcomes of Cancer Patients Undergoing Percutaneous Pericardiocentesis for Pericardial Effusion. J Am Coll Cardiol. 2015 Sep 8;66(10):1119-28. doi: 10.1016/j.jacc.2015.06.1332. Erratum in: J Am Coll Cardiol. 2015 Nov 17;66(20):2269. PMID: 26337990; PMCID: PMC4560839.

47. A 65-year-old male with stable coronary artery disease is treated with cabozantinib for renal cell carcinoma. He is also on aspirin 81 mg daily and atorvastatin 80 mg daily. During his follow up appointment, his blood pressure is 160/86 mmHg.

He denied having any symptoms. Of the following, what is the best way to manage his hypertension?

A. Begin an angiotensin-converting enzyme (ACE) inhibitor and continue cabozantinib
B. Begin diltiazem and continue cabozantinib without interruption
C. Begin verapamil, hold cabozantinib and resume when the blood pressure is within normal range
D. Stop cabozantinib and consider a different treatment for renal cell carcinoma

A pooled analysis of patients with metastatic renal cell carcinoma treated on phase II and III clinical trials was conducted to evaluate the impact of angiotensin system inhibitors (ASI) on outcomes. A total of 4,736 patients were included, of whom 1,487 received ASIs and 783 received other antihypertensive agents. For the overall cohort, overall survival was significantly longer in ASI users compared with users of other antihypertensive agents (adjusted hazard ratio [HR], 0.838; 95% confidence interval [CI], 0.731 – 0.960; $p = 0.0105$). Progression-free survival was also significantly longer in ASI users. When stratified by type of therapy, a benefit in overall survival was observed in ASI users compared with nonusers in those receiving VEGF therapy, but not temsirolimus or IFNα.

Although calcium-channel blockers have been shown to be effective in controlling anti-VEGF tyrosine kinase-related hypertension, diltiazem and verapamil both interact with cabozantinib, and may increase cabozantinib levels. Cabozantinib is associated with several adverse reactions including, but not limited to, hemorrhage, arterial and venous thromboembolic events, and hypertensive crisis.

Reference(s):

- McKay RR, Rodriguez GE, Lin X, Kaymakcalan MD, Hamnvik OP, Sabbisetti VS, Bhatt RS, Simantov R, Choueiri TK. Angiotensin system inhibitors and survival outcomes in patients with metastatic renal cell carcinoma. Clin Cancer Res. 2015 Jun 1;21(11):2471-9. doi: 10.1158/1078-0432.CCR-14-2332. Epub 2015 Feb 27. PMID: 25724518; PMCID: PMC4566854.
- Waliany S, Sainani KL, Park LS, Zhang CA, Srinivas S, Witteles RM. Increase in Blood Pressure Associated With Tyrosine Kinase Inhibitors Targeting Vascular Endothelial Growth Factor. JACC CardioOncol. 2019 Sep 24;1(1):24-36. doi: 10.1016/j.jaccao.2019.08.012. PMID: 34396159; PMCID: PMC8352203.

48. Immune checkpoint blocking antibodies increase anti-tumor immunity by:

A. Activating normal co-inhibitory molecules on T cells
B. Activating normal co-stimulatory molecules on T cells
C. Inhibiting normal co-inhibitory molecules on T cells
D. Inhibiting normal co-stimulatory molecules on T cells

Reference(s):

- Jacob JB, Jacob MK, Parajuli P. Review of immune checkpoint inhibitors in immuno-oncology. Adv Pharmacol. 2021;91:111-139. doi: 10.1016/bs.apha.2021.01.002. Epub 2021 May 20. PMID: 34099106.

49. Which of the following is a potential complication seen in patients with acute promyelocytic leukemia treated with all-trans retinoic acid and/or arsenic trioxide?

    A. Differentiation syndrome

    B. Hemophagocytic lymphohistiocytosis (HLH)

    C. Macrophage activation syndrome

    D. Trousseau syndrome

Reference(s):

- Sanz MA, Montesinos P. How we prevent and treat differentiation syndrome in patients with acute promyelocytic leukemia. Blood. 2014 May 1;123(18):2777-82. doi: 10.1182/blood-2013-10-512640. Epub 2014 Mar 13. PMID: 24627526.
- Stahl M, Tallman MS. Differentiation syndrome in acute promyelocytic leukaemia. Br J Haematol. 2019 Oct;187(2):157-162. doi: 10.1111/bjh.16151. Epub 2019 Aug 13. PMID: 31410848.

50. Which of the following screening biomarkers has been shown to have both diagnostic and prognostic significance for cardiac involvement in patients with carcinoid heart disease?

    A. Activin A

    B. Cardiac troponin T

    C. Chromogranin A

    D. N-terminal pro-B-type natriuretic peptide (NT-proBNP)

    Carcinoid heart disease is one of the several complications that may affect patients with carcinoid syndrome. Although its pathophysiology is not completely understood, chronic exposure to excessive circulating serotonin (5-hydroxytryptamine) is considered a contributing factor to carcinoid heart disease. This is characterized by the development of plaque-like, fibrous endocardial thickening mainly involving the right heart and affecting the pulmonic and tricuspid valves. The presence of carcinoid heart disease represents an independent negative prognostic factor in patients with advanced neuroendocrine tumors. Having sensitive and specific biomarkers that can diagnose and predict the severity of carcinoid heart disease would allow better monitoring of these patients. NT-proBNP and chromogranin A have been identified as useful diagnostic markers in patients with carcinoid heart disease. However, compared to chromogranin A levels alone, the combination of elevated NT-proBNP and chromogranin A have been shown to provide better prognostic information regarding overall survival.

Reference(s):

- Davar J, Connolly HM, Caplin ME, Pavel M, Zacks J, Bhattacharyya S, Cuthbertson DJ, Dobson R, Grozinsky-Glasberg S, Steeds RP, Dreyfus G, Pellikka PA, Toumpanakis C. Diagnosing and Managing Carcinoid Heart Disease in Patients With Neuroendocrine Tumors: An Expert Statement. J Am Coll Cardiol. 2017 Mar 14;69(10):1288-1304. doi: 10.1016/j.jacc.2016.12.030. PMID: 28279296.

- Korse CM, Taal BG, de Groot CA, Bakker RH, Bonfrer JM. Chromogranin-A and N-terminal pro-brain natriuretic peptide: an excellent pair of biomarkers for diagnostics in patients with neuroendocrine tumor. J Clin Oncol. 2009 Sep 10;27(26):4293-9. doi: 10.1200/JCO.2008.18.7047. Epub 2009 Aug 10. PMID: 19667278.

51. A 48-year-old female with metastatic neuroendocrine intestinal tumor is being evaluated for liver transplantation. She has New York Heart Association class 3 symptoms and a heart failure hospitalization in the past 6 months. Transthoracic echocardiogram showed mild right ventricular hypertrophy, thickened and restricted tricuspid valve leaflets that failed to coapt, severe tricuspid regurgitation, and evidence of a thickened pulmonary valve with severe regurgitation. The patient is currently on furosemide, spironolactone, and octreotide. What is the best next step in the cardiovascular management of this patient?

    A. Proceed with liver transplantation and repeat an echocardiogram in 6 months
    B. Referral for heart transplantation prior to liver transplantation
    C. Tricuspid and pulmonary valve replacement prior to liver transplantation
    D. Tricuspid valve replacement prior to liver transplantation

    There is limited evidence on the management of patients with carcinoid heart disease (CHD) and valvular dysfunction requiring non-cardiac surgery such as hepatic lesion resection or liver transplantation. Nonetheless, determining optimal timing for cardiac surgery in these patients is complicated due to the complexity of their condition.

    In a study, 14 patients with earlier valve replacement for CHD were compared to 28 carcinoid patients without CHD. All patients had hepatic resection for metastatic carcinoid disease and carcinoid syndrome. There was no operative mortality, and there was no statistical difference in operative complications such as operative blood loss and cardiorespiratory events. Symptom-free survival for CHD and non-CHD groups was 69% and 81% at 1 year ($p = 0.22$) and 61% and 44% ($p = 0.17$) at 5 years, respectively. Overall survival CHD and non-CHD groups was 100% at 1 year and 100% and 70% ($p = 0.002$) at 5 years.

    Another study sought to identify factors that might be associated with early mortality rates and late outcomes. The authors analyzed 240 adult patients who underwent surgery for carcinoid heart disease at the Mayo Clinic between November 1985 and January 2018. Before surgery, 157 patients (70%) had NYHA class III or IV symptoms. Between 1985 and 1994, early mortality was 29%, and it decreased to 7% between 1995 and 2004, and has been 5% since that time (for the rest of the patients who underwent surgery). Overall survival estimates at 1, 3, and 5 years were 69%, 48%, and 34%, respectively. Increased early mortality was associated with older age and worse NYHA class at presentation.

Reference(s):

- Askew JW, Connolly HM. Carcinoid valve disease. Curr Treat Options Cardiovasc Med. 2013 Oct;15(5):544-55. doi: 10.1007/s11936-013-0265-2. PMID: 23955119.
- Davar J, Connolly HM, Caplin ME, Pavel M, Zacks J, Bhattacharyya S, Cuthbertson DJ, Dobson R, Grozinsky-Glasberg S, Steeds RP, Dreyfus G, Pellikka

PA, Toumpanakis C. Diagnosing and Managing Carcinoid Heart Disease in Patients With Neuroendocrine Tumors: An Expert Statement. J Am Coll Cardiol. 2017 Mar 14;69(10):1288-1304. doi: 10.1016/j.jacc.2016.12.030. PMID: 28279296.

- Lillegard JB, Fisher JE, Mckenzie TJ, Que FG, Farnell MB, Kendrick ML, Donohue JH, Reid-Lombardo K, Schaff HV, Connolly HM, Nagorney DM. Hepatic resection for the carcinoid syndrome in patients with severe carcinoid heart disease: does valve replacement permit safe hepatic resection? J Am Coll Surg. 2011 Jul;213(1):130-6; discussion 136-8. doi: 10.1016/j.jamcollsurg.2011.03.029. Epub 2011 Apr 13. PMID: 21493110.
- Nguyen A, Schaff HV, Abel MD, Luis SA, Lahr BD, Halfdanarson TR, Connolly HM. Improving outcome of valve replacement for carcinoid heart disease. J Thorac Cardiovasc Surg. 2019 Jul;158(1):99-107.e2. doi: 10.1016/j.jtcvs.2018.09.025. Epub 2018 Oct 3. PMID: 30527716.

52. Which of the following statements is correct about carriers of clonal hematopoiesis of indeterminate potential (CHIP)?

    A. CHIP confers a 4-fold increased risk of myocardial infarction.

    B. Individuals with CHIP have a 5% increase in all-cause mortality.

    C. The diagnosis of CHIP requires the presence of definitive morphological evidence of a hematologic neoplasm.

    D. The risk of developing a hematologic malignancy is greater than 1% per year.

    A study using participants from four case-control studies (4,726 participants with coronary artery disease and 3,529 controls) investigated the association between CHIP and coronary artery disease, and causality by using atherosclerosis-prone mice. The analysis revealed that carriers of CHIP had a risk of coronary artery disease that was 1.9 times as great as non-carriers (95% confidence interval [CI], 1.4 – 2.7) and a risk of myocardial infarction that was 4 times as great as in non-carriers (95% CI, 2.4 – 6.7). Tet2 knockout mice were also shown to have evidence of accelerated atherosclerosis.

Reference(s):

- Jaiswal S, Natarajan P, Silver AJ, Gibson CJ, Bick AG, Shvartz E, McConkey M, Gupta N, Gabriel S, Ardissino D, Baber U, Mehran R, Fuster V, Danesh J, Frossard P, Saleheen D, Melander O, Sukhova GK, Neuberg D, Libby P, Kathiresan S, Ebert BL. Clonal Hematopoiesis and Risk of Atherosclerotic Cardiovascular Disease. N Engl J Med. 2017 Jul 13;377(2):111-121. doi: 10.1056/NEJMoa1701719. Epub 2017 Jun 21. PMID: 28636844; PMCID: PMC6717509.

53. A 35-year-old female with history of childhood Hodgkin's lymphoma presents to her follow-up appointment for chronic systolic heart failure due to chemotherapy-induced cardiomyopathy (CCMP). Her left ventricular ejection fraction is 20% and she continues to experience New York Heart Association class 4 symptoms. Which of the following statements is most accurate in patients with CCMP undergoing heart transplantation?

    A. CCMP patients are more likely to require biventricular support before heart transplantation than patients with other non-ischemic cardiomyopathies.

B. CCMP patients have worse survival after heart transplantation than patients with other non-ischemic cardiomyopathies.

C. CCMP patients tend to have more co-morbidities compared to other non-ischemic cardiomyopathy patients.

D. The incidence of infection after heart transplantation is similar to patients with other forms of non-ischemic cardiomyopathy.

In a retrospective study (using the International Society of Heart and Lung Transplantation Registry), Oliveira et al reported on the short- and long-term post-transplant outcomes in patients with CCMP. Two hundred and thirty-two patients with CCMP were compared to 8,890 patients with a non-ischemic cardiomyopathy (NICMP). The analysis showed that survival at 1, 3, and 5 years was similar between the groups ($p = 0.19$). Compared with NICMP patients, CCMP patients had a higher rate of post-transplant infection (22% vs 14%, $p = 0.004$) and malignancies (5% vs 2%, $p = 0.006$), but neither affected survival. Interestingly, patients with CCMP were twice as likely as those with NICMP to require right ventricular assist devices (RVAD) before heart transplantation (5.6% vs 2.3%, $p = 0.0021$). This is the basis for answer choice A, but we recognize that there is limited data on this topic and this may change in the future.

Moreover, there has been at least 2 studies (using the INTERMACS registry) addressing the use of mechanical circulatory support (MCS) in patients with CCMP. In 2014, Oliveira et al published a retrospective study on the use of durable MCS in this patient population and found that compared with patients with NICMP, those with CCMP had MCS more often implanted as destination therapy, required more right ventricular assist device support, and had a higher risk of bleeding. A more contemporary analysis by Guha et al on the outcomes in patients with CCMP undergoing left ventricular assist device implantation showed similar survival between patients with CCMP and those with ischemic or dilated cardiomyopathy. In addition, only 5 patients with CCMP (1.6%) required right ventricular support in the first week, compared with 103 (1.2%) with dilated cardiomyopathy and 27 (2%) with ischemic cardiomyopathy. Of note, patients with history of RVAD or requiring concomitant RVAD implantation were excluded.

Ramu et al recently published a study on heart transplantation in patients with Adriamycin-associated cardiomyopathy (ACM). The authors used the United Network for Organ Sharing database from 2008 to 2018. Their analysis demonstrated that patients with ACM were less often treated with a left ventricular assist device as a bridge to heart transplantation. They speculate this may be related to the aforementioned study from Oliveira et al in 2014 showing a greater need for RVAD in this population. Further research in this area is greatly needed.

Reference(s):

- Guha A, Caraballo C, Jain P, Miller PE, Owusu-Guha J, Clark KAA, Velazquez EJ, Ahmad T, Baldassarre LA, Addison D, Weintraub NL, Desai NR. Outcomes in patients with anthracycline-induced cardiomyopathy undergoing left ventricular assist devices implantation. ESC Heart Fail. 2021 Aug;8(4):2866-2875. doi: 10.1002/ehf2.13362. Epub 2021 May 13. PMID: 33982867; PMCID: PMC8318466.

- Oliveira GH, Dupont M, Naftel D, Myers SL, Yuan Y, Tang WH, Gonzalez-Stawinski G, Young JB, Taylor DO, Starling RC. Increased need for right ventricular support in patients with chemotherapy-induced cardiomyopathy undergoing mechanical circulatory support: outcomes from the INTERMACS Registry (Interagency Registry for Mechanically Assisted Circulatory Support). J Am Coll Cardiol. 2014 Jan 28;63(3):240-8. doi: 10.1016/j.jacc.2013.09.040. Epub 2013 Oct 23. PMID: 24161324.
- Oliveira GH, Hardaway BW, Kucheryavaya AY, Stehlik J, Edwards LB, Taylor DO. Characteristics and survival of patients with chemotherapy-induced cardiomyopathy undergoing heart transplantation. J Heart Lung Transplant. 2012 Aug;31(8):805-10. doi: 10.1016/j.healun.2012.03.018. Epub 2012 May 1. PMID: 22551930.
- Ramu B, Masotti M, Tedford RJ, Cogswell RJ. Heart Transplantation in Adriamycin-Associated Cardiomyopathy in the Contemporary Era of Advanced Heart Failure Therapies. JACC CardioOncol. 2021 Jun 15;3(2):294-301. doi: 10.1016/j.jaccao.2021.02.010. PMID: 34396337; PMCID: PMC8352281.

54. A 65-year-old female with leiomyosarcoma of the uterus is diagnosed with acute deep vein thrombosis (DVT) of the right lower extremity. She has completed 7 months of anticoagulation with rivaroxaban 20 mg daily without complications. A month ago, she started to notice swelling in the left lower extremity while on rivaroxaban. An ultrasound shows a new DVT in that extremity. What is the best next step in the management of DVT in this patient?

    A. Change rivaroxaban to warfarin

    B. Change rivaroxaban to low-molecular-weight heparin

    C. Continue rivaroxaban for at least 6 more months

    D. Discontinue rivaroxaban and insert a vena cava filter

    In cases of suspected treatment failure, it is important to assess for compliance with anticoagulant therapy and appropriate dosing of the agent as well as for other causes of hypercoagulability (e.g., antiphospholipid syndrome). In addition, residual DVT should be excluded. In this case, the patient developed a DVT in the contralateral lower extremity after 7 months of anticoagulation. One way to confirm compliance with treatment is to contact the patient's pharmacy and confirm the number of dispenses for the given medication. If treatment failure is confirmed, full dose low-molecular-weight heparin (LMWH) is recommended for at least 4 weeks.

Reference(s):

- Rodger MA, Miranda S, Delluc A, Carrier M. Management of suspected and confirmed recurrent venous thrombosis while on anticoagulant therapy. What next? Thromb Res. 2019 Aug;180:105-109. doi: 10.1016/j.thromres.2019.06.017. Epub 2019 Jun 26. PMID: 31279158.
- Schulman S. How I treat recurrent venous thromboembolism in patients receiving anticoagulant therapy. Blood. 2017 Jun 22;129(25):3285-3293. doi: 10.1182/blood-2017-03-742304. Epub 2017 May 8. PMID: 28483766.

55. Which of the following statements is most accurate about the long-term use of a vena cava filter in the management of venous thromboembolism (VTE) in patients with cancer?

A. A permanent filter is preferred in patients with cancer.

B. It has been shown to decrease the risk of pulmonary embolism.

C. It improves survival.

D. It is associated with an increased long-term risk for lower extremity thrombus.

A retrospective observational study including 96 patients with inferior vena cava filters (IVCF) who had a contrast-enhanced CT scan of the abdomen at a minimum of 4 years post-IVCF implantation showed an overall rate of filter fracture of 14% and partial/complete IVC occlusion of 13% (7.3% total and 5.2% partial). IVC perforation rates were higher among retrievable filters (70%) compared with permanent devices (15%) ($p < 0.0001$). Another analysis reported additional complications such as embolization and recurrent VTE.

Reference(s):

- Ayad MT, Gillespie DL. Long-term complications of inferior vena cava filters. J Vasc Surg Venous LymphatDisord. 2019 Jan;7(1):139-144. doi: 10.1016/j.jvsv.2018.01.022. Epub 2018 Aug 17. PMID: 30126794.
- Wang SL, Siddiqui A, Rosenthal E. Long-term complications of inferior vena cava filters. J Vasc Surg Venous LymphatDisord. 2017 Jan;5(1):33-41. doi: 10.1016/j.jvsv.2016.07.002. Epub 2016 Sep 26. PMID: 27987607.

56. Which of the following criteria are the principal determinants defining the severity of cytokine release syndrome?

A. Fever and arthralgia

B. Fever and coagulopathy

C. Hypotension and hypoxia

D. Pleural effusion and tachycardia

2018 ASBMT Consensus Grading for Cytokine Release Syndrome and Neurological Toxicity

CRS Criteria	Grade 1	Grade 2	Grade 3	Grade 4
Fever	≥38°C	≥38°C	≥38°C	≥38°C
Hypotension	None	No vasopressor	1 vasopressor with or without vasopressin	Multiple vasopressors (excluding vasopressin)
Hypoxia	None	Low-flow nasal cannula or blow-by oxygen	High-flow nasal cannula, facemask, non-rebreather mas, or Venturia mask	Positive pressure ventilation (e.g., CPAP, BiPAP, intubation, mechanical ventilation)
Grade 5 – Death				

Reference(s):

- Lee DW, Santomasso BD, Locke FL, Ghobadi A, Turtle CJ, Brudno JN, Maus MV, Park JH, Mead E, Pavletic S, Go WY, Eldjerou L, Gardner RA, Frey N, Curran KJ, Peggs K, Pasquini M, DiPersio JF, van den Brink MRM, Komanduri KV, Grupp SA, Neelapu SS. ASTCT Consensus Grading for Cytokine Release Syndrome and Neurologic Toxicity Associated with Immune Effector Cells. Biol Blood Marrow Transplant. 2019 Apr;25(4):625-638. doi: 10.1016/j.bbmt.2018.12.758. Epub 2018 Dec 25. PMID: 30592986.
- Riegler LL, Jones GP, Lee DW. Current approaches in the grading and management of cytokine release syndrome after chimeric antigen receptor T-cell therapy. Ther Clin Risk Manag. 2019 Feb 28;15:323-335. doi: 10.2147/TCRM.S150524. PMID: 30880998; PMCID: PMC6400118.
- Shimabukuro-Vornhagen A, Gödel P, Subklewe M, Stemmler HJ, Schlößer HA, Schlaak M, Kochanek M, Böll B, von Bergwelt-Baildon MS. Cytokine release syndrome. J Immunother Cancer. 2018 Jun 15;6(1):56. doi: 10.1186/s40425-018-0343-9. PMID: 29907163; PMCID: PMC6003181.

57. A 68-year-old female with uterine cancer presents with worsening left lower extremity swelling and tenderness over the past 2 weeks. There is evidence of skin ulceration and venous engorgement. A venous ultrasound shows an acute thrombus in the common femoral vein. What is the best next step in the management of this patient?

    A. Initiate dabigatran and repeat a venous ultrasound in 3 months

    B. Initiate aspirin and warfarin and repeat a venous ultrasound in 3 months

    C. Initiate low-molecular-weight heparin and consider percutaneous mechanical thrombectomy

    D. Place an inferior vena cava filter and reassess in 3 months

    Iliofemoral deep vein thrombosis (DVT) is associated with an increased risk of embolism and post-thrombotic complications. A significant number of patients with iliofemoral DVT develop post-thrombotic syndrome, which can result in venous claudication, edema, and limb ischemia. Phlegmasia cerulea dolens is a severe complication that can result in limb amputation and death. In addition to treatment with full anticoagulation, patients with evidence of limb complication as this patient should also be considered for mechanical or catheter-directed thrombolysis. A multidisciplinary approach consisting of vascular surgeons, interventional radiologists, cardiologists, and in this case, oncology is recommended.

Reference(s):

- Liu D, Peterson E, Dooner J, Baerlocher M, Zypchen L, Gagnon J, Delorme M, Sing CK, Wong J, Guzman R, Greenfield G, Moodley O, Yenson P; Interdisciplinary Expert Panel on Iliofemoral Deep Vein Thrombosis (InterEPID). Diagnosis and management of iliofemoral deep vein thrombosis: clinical practice guideline. CMAJ. 2015 Nov 17;187(17):1288-1296. doi: 10.1503/cmaj.141614. Epub 2015 Sep 28. PMID: 26416989; PMCID: PMC4646749.

58. A 59-year-old male with metastatic neuroendocrine tumor with primary involvement of the liver presents with worsening lower extremity edema and pain. The patient had undergone extensive evaluation with multiple venous ultrasounds showing no evidence of deep vein thrombosis. A transthoracic echocardiogram showed normal left ventricular function and no valve disease. N-terminal pro-brain natriuretic peptide (NT-proBNP) is normal. What is the next best step in the management of this patient?

A. Obtain a cardiac MRI

B. Obtain a CT scan with contrast of the chest, abdomen, and pelvis

C. Recommend wearing compression stockings

D. Start furosemide and repeat a venous ultrasound

In this patient, evaluation for inferior vena cava (IVC) syndrome due to external compression from his liver mass(es) and/or lymphatic drainage problem should be considered. Given his known liver process, a CT scan with intravenous contrast of the chest, abdomen, and pelvis would help evaluate for IVC syndrome due to tumor compression. Obstruction of the IVC is typically caused by a primary thrombotic event, which can be congenital or acquired. In this case, a congenital etiology is less likely given the acuity of his symptoms. A normal transthoracic echocardiogram and NT-proBNP essentially exclude heart failure.

Reference(s):

- McAree BJ, O'Donnell ME, Fitzmaurice GJ, Reid JA, Spence RA, Lee B. Inferior vena cava thrombosis: a review of current practice. Vasc Med. 2013 Feb;18(1):32-43. doi: 10.1177/1358863X12471967. PMID: 23439778.
- Lawrensia S, Khan YS. Inferior Vena Cava Syndrome. 2022 Jul 12. In: StatPearls [Internet]. Treasure Island (FL): StatPearls Publishing; 2022 Jan–. PMID: 32809720.

59. A 57-year-old male with metastatic adenocarcinoma of the esophagus presents with worsening dyspnea on exertion and atrial fibrillation with rapid ventricular response. A transthoracic echocardiogram revealed right ventricular dilation with free wall hypokinesis and apical sparing. A chest CT scan demonstrates extensive bilateral pulmonary emboli and a large thrombus within the right atrium. Blood pressure is 90/50 mmHg and heart rate is 110 beats per minute. In addition to starting anticoagulation, what is the next best step to consider in the management of this patient?

A. Cardiac catheterization with coronary angiogram

B. Evaluate for thrombectomy

C. Systemic thrombolysis

D. Transesophageal echocardiogram and possible direct-current cardioversion

This patient has a significant thrombus burden and is at risk for recurrent pulmonary embolism. He has evidence of right ventricular dilation and dysfunction, is hypotensive, and tachycardic. He may also require to continue on potentially life-prolonging or palliative chemotherapy for his cancer. This should be considered a massive pulmonary embolism and be treated with thrombectomy in addition to anticoagulation as tolerated. Thrombectomy or thrombolysis can be achieved in different ways including systemic thrombolysis, catheter-directed thrombolysis, percutaneous mechanical or pharmacomechanical intervention, and surgical embolectomy. The choice of treatment modality will depend on the patient's condition and expertise available at the treating institution.

Reference(s):

- Moriarty JM, Edwards M, Plotnik AN. Intervention in Massive Pulmonary Embolus: Catheter Thrombectomy/Thromboaspiration versus Systemic Lysis versus Surgical Thrombectomy. Semin InterventRadiol. 2018 Jun;35(2):108-115. doi: 10.1055/s-0038-1642039. Epub 2018 Jun 4. PMID: 29872246; PMCID: PMC5986563.

60. A 70-year-old female presents with worsening fatigue and dyspnea on exertion. She was diagnosed with desmoid fibromatosis and was started on sorafenib. She has history of Hodgkin lymphoma 30 years ago treated with non-anthracycline containing chemotherapy and no radiation therapy per patient's wishes. She has history of mitral valve disease requiring replacement with a bioprosthetic valve one year ago. Vital signs in clinic showed a pulse of 61 beats per minute (bpm), blood pressure of 120/60 mmHg, respiratory rate of 12 breaths per minute, and oxygen saturation on room air of 99%. Physical examination revealed an irregularly irregular rhythm, holosystolic murmur at the left lower sternal border, and normal jugular venous pressure. Electrocardiogram demonstrated atrial fibrillation with a heart rate of 60 bpm. What is the best next step in the management of this patient?

    A. Dobutamine stress echocardiogram
    B. Cardiac catheterization with coronary angiography
    C. Transesophageal echocardiogram with possible direct-current cardioversion
    D. Transthoracic echocardiogram with Doppler

    Transthoracic echocardiography would be the preliminary investigation both to assess the mitral valve and to assess the left ventricular function. The information obtained would determine the next management steps, which could include a transesophageal echocardiogram and coronary angiogram. Dobutamine stress echocardiogram should be avoided due to atrial fibrillation.

Reference(s):

- Lancellotti P, Pibarot P, Chambers J, Edvardsen T, Delgado V, Dulgheru R, Pepi M, Cosyns B, Dweck MR, Garbi M, Magne J, Nieman K, Rosenhek R, Bernard A, Lowenstein J, Vieira ML, Rabischoffsky A, Vyhmeister RH, Zhou X, Zhang Y, Zamorano JL, Habib G. Recommendations for the imaging assessment of prosthetic heart valves: a report from the European Association of Cardiovascular Imaging endorsed by the Chinese Society of Echocardiography, the Inter-American Society of Echocardiography, and the Brazilian Department of Cardiovascular Imaging. Eur Heart J Cardiovasc Imaging. 2016 Jun;17(6):589-90. doi: 10.1093/ehjci/jew025. Epub 2016 May 3. PMID: 27143783.

61. A 25-year-old male with history of Hodgkin's lymphoma at the age of 12 years was referred to your clinic for cardiovascular surveillance. His cancer treatment included four cycles of ABVE (doxorubicin with cumulative dose of 200 mg/m2, bleomycin, vincristine, and etoposide) and mantle radiation. He denies having any symptoms at this time and his vital signs are within normal range. A thyroid ultrasound showed a right-sided 2-centimeter solid, hypoechoic nodule. Fine-needle aspiration demonstrated atypia of undetermined significance. What is the best next step in the management of this patient?

A. Perform a PET-CT scan

B. Referral for hemithyroidectomy for excision

C. Repeat a thyroid ultrasound in 12 months

D. Repeat a thyroid ultrasound in 6 months

A multicenter study evaluated the long-term risk of thyroid cancer associated with radiation treatment among 12,547 5-year survivors of a childhood cancer diagnosed between 1970 and 1986 in the Childhood Cancer Survivor Study (using the most recent cohort follow-up to 2005 based on the time of this analysis). The authors found that the risk of thyroid cancer increased linearly with radiation dose up to about 20 Gy. At thyroid radiation doses >20 Gy, a downturn in the dose-response relationship was observed. Age exposure, female gender, and time since exposure were identified as risk factors.

In a nested case-control study, 69 cases with pathologically confirmed thyroid cancer and 265 matched controls without thyroid cancer were identified from 14,054 5-year survivors of cancer during childhood from the Childhood Cancer Survivor Study cohort. The risk of thyroid cancer increased with radiation doses up to 20-29 Gy (odds ratio, 9.8; 95 confidence interval [CI], 3.2-34.8). Twenty-nine (42%) cases had a first diagnosis of Hodgkin lymphoma compared with 49 (19%) controls. Eleven (42%) of those who had Hodgkin lymphoma had subsequent thyroid cancers smaller than 1 cm compared with 6 (17%) of those who had other types of childhood cancer ($p = 0.07$).

Data from the British Childhood Cancer Survivors Study showed that the risk of thyroid cancer was highest after Hodgkin lymphoma (relative risk [RR], 3.3; 95% CI, 1.1 - 10.1) and non-Hodgkin lymphoma (RR 3.4; 95% CI 1.1 - 10.7) relative to leukemia (RR 1.0) ($p < 0.001$). Survivors treated with radiotherapy in childhood had a RR of 4.6 (95% CI, 1.4 – 15.1) relative to survivors not treated with radiotherapy ($p = 0.003$).

Reference(s):

- Bhatti P, Veiga LH, Ronckers CM, Sigurdson AJ, Stovall M, Smith SA, Weathers R, Leisenring W, Mertens AC, Hammond S, Friedman DL, Neglia JP, Meadows AT, Donaldson SS, Sklar CA, Robison LL, Inskip PD. Risk of second primary thyroid cancer after radiotherapy for a childhood cancer in a large cohort study: an update from the childhood cancer survivor study. Radiat Res. 2010 Dec;174(6):741-52. doi: 10.1667/RR2240.1. Epub 2010 Oct 6. PMID: 21128798; PMCID: PMC3080023.

- Sigurdson AJ, Ronckers CM, Mertens AC, Stovall M, Smith SA, Liu Y, Berkow RL, Hammond S, Neglia JP, Meadows AT, Sklar CA, Robison LL, Inskip PD. Primary thyroid cancer after a first tumour in childhood (the Childhood Cancer Survivor Study): a nested case-control study. Lancet. 2005 Jun 11-17;365(9476):2014-23. doi: 10.1016/S0140-6736(05)66695-0. PMID: 15950715.
- Taylor AJ, Croft AP, Palace AM, Winter DL, Reulen RC, Stiller CA, Stevens MC, Hawkins MM. Risk of thyroid cancer in survivors of childhood cancer: results from the British Childhood Cancer Survivor Study. Int J Cancer. 2009 Nov 15;125(10):2400-5. doi: 10.1002/ijc.24581. PMID: 19610069.

62. A 61-year-old male with chronic systolic heart failure with a left ventricular ejection fraction less than 20% and normal right ventricular size and function has been diagnosed with prostate adenocarcinoma (Gleason grade 3+4 = 7 on the right and Gleason grade 4+3 = 7 on the left). His most recent prostate-specific antigen (PSA) is 80 ng/mL, previously 40 ng/mL two months ago. Bone scintigraphy shows no evidence of osseous metastatic disease. He is now admitted for the fourth time with acute on chronic systolic heart failure requiring inotropic therapy with dobutamine. What is the most reasonable next step in the management of this patient?

    A. Discharge home on palliative dobutamine
    B. Referral for heart transplantation
    C. Referral for left ventricular assist device and start prostate cancer therapy
    D. Referral to hospice

    Prostate cancer therapy needs to be safely started in this patient. This requires stabilization of his heart failure. He would not be a candidate for heart transplantation given his ongoing cancer and as such the most suitable approach would be to consider left ventricular assist device (LVAD) therapy in this stage of heart failure.

    A recent retrospective study published in JACC CardioOncology analyzed data from 2 tertiary heart failure and oncology programs in the United States. Using the INTERMACS database, among 1,123 patients who underwent LVAD implantation between 2005 and 2019, 22 patients with LVAD and active cancer and 66 matched non-cancer controls were identified. Prostate cancer was the most common malignancy. There was no significant difference in unadjusted Kaplan-Meier medial survival estimates from the time of LVAD implantation between patients with cancer (3.53 years; 95% confidence interval [CI], 1.41 – 5.33) and non-cancer patients (3.03 years; 95% CI, 1.03 – 4.12; $p = 0.04$). Interestingly, patients with cancer had less gastrointestinal bleeding compared with those without cancer. Other complications, including LVAD thrombosis, stroke, and infection, were not statistically different.

Reference(s):

- Heidenreich PA, Bozkurt B, Aguilar D, Allen LA, Byun JJ, Colvin MM, Deswal A, Drazner MH, Dunlay SM, Evers LR, Fang JC, Fedson SE, Fonarow GC, Hayek SS, Hernandez AF, Khazanie P, Kittleson MM, Lee CS, Link MS, Milano CA,

Nnacheta LC, Sandhu AT, Stevenson LW, Vardeny O, Vest AR, Yancy CW. 2022 AHA/ACC/HFSA Guideline for the Management of Heart Failure: Executive Summary: A Report of the American College of Cardiology/American Heart Association Joint Committee on Clinical Practice Guidelines. J Am Coll Cardiol. 2022 May 3;79(17):1757-1780. doi: 10.1016/j.jacc.2021.12.011. Epub 2022 Apr 1. PMID: 35379504.

- Schlam I, Lee AY, Li S, Sheikh FH, Zaghlol R, Basyal B, Gallagher C, Molina E, Mahr C, Cheng RK, Barac A. Left Ventricular Assist Devices in Patients With Active Malignancies. JACC CardioOncol. 2021 Jun 15;3(2):305-315. doi: 10.1016/j.jaccao.2021.04.008. PMID: 34396339; PMCID: PMC8352017.

63. A 60-year-old male with a large right hilar/suprahilar pulmonary mass invading the mediastinum presents with recurrent headaches and swelling of the face and upper extremities. Vital signs showed a pulse of 108 beats per minute (bpm), blood pressure of 89/55 mmHg, respiratory rate of 16 breaths per minute, and oxygen saturation on room air 98%. What is the most likely diagnosis?

    A. Acute coronary syndrome
    B. Acute pulmonary embolism
    C. Cardiac tamponade
    D. Superior vena cava syndrome

    Superior vena cava syndrome can be the initial presentation in 60% of undiagnosed tumors. These tumors are usually lung cancer or non-Hodgkin lymphoma (85-90% of cases) with the remainder being metastatic cancers.

Reference(s):

- Patriarcheas V, Grammoustianou M, Ptohis N, Thanou I, Kostis M, Gkiozos I, Charpidou A, Trontzas I, Syrigos N, Kotteas E, Dimakakos E. Malignant Superior Vena Cava Syndrome: State of the Art. Cureus. 2022 Jan 4;14(1):e20924. doi: 10.7759/cureus.20924. PMID: 35004083; PMCID: PMC8727327.

64. What is the most appropriate therapeutic intervention to address the diagnosis in Question 63?

    A. Endovascular recanalization with or without stenting
    B. High-dose intravenous steroids
    C. Radiation therapy
    D. Systemic thrombolytic therapy

    Endovascular recanalization is the fastest way to alleviate symptoms (usually within 0-72 hours compared to radiotherapy where it can take up to 2 weeks). The efficacy is also higher (95-100%) compared to radiotherapy (80%).

Reference(s):

- Watkinson AF, Yeow TN, Fraser C. Endovascular stenting to treat obstruction of the superior vena cava. BMJ. 2008 Jun 21;336(7658):1434-7. doi: 10.1136/bmj.39562.512789.80. PMID: 18566082; PMCID: PMC2432169.

65. A 67-year-old male with essential hypertension and asymptomatic paroxysmal atrial fibrillation is diagnosed with mantle cell lymphoma. In addition to easy bruising, he also has intermittent nausea. His oncologist recommends treatment with ibrutinib. Due to the potential for drug-drug interaction, which of the following medications should be avoided when a patient is taking ibrutinib?

A. Amlodipine

B. Diltiazem

C. Metoprolol

D. Prochlorperazine (Compazine)

As diltiazem is a moderate inhibitor of CYP3A4 and ibrutinib is a substrate of this enzyme, prolonged co-administration of the two drugs is likely to result in reduced ibrutinib clearance and subsequent cardiotoxicity and potentially even death.

Reference(s):

- Falconer N, Ryan M, Badman B, Carrington C. Death from diltiazem-ibrutinib interaction. Aust Prescr. 2021 Jun;44(3):107-108. doi: 10.18773/austprescr.2021.019. Epub 2021 Jun 1. PMID: 34211249; PMCID: PMC8236876.
- Ganatra S, Sharma A, Shah S, Chaudhry GM, Martin DT, Neilan TG, Mahmood SS, Barac A, Groarke JD, Hayek SS, Dani S, Venesy D, Patten R, Nohria A. Ibrutinib-Associated Atrial Fibrillation. JACC Clin Electrophysiol. 2018 Dec;4(12):1491-1500. doi: 10.1016/j.jacep.2018.06.004. Epub 2018 Aug 29. PMID: 30573111.
- Stühlinger MC, Weltermann A, Staber P, Heintel D, Nösslinger T, Steurer M. Recommendations for ibrutinib treatment in patients with atrial fibrillation and/or elevated cardiovascular risk. Wien KlinWochenschr. 2020 Feb;132(3-4):97-109. doi: 10.1007/s00508-019-1534-1. Epub 2019 Aug 14. PMID: 31414181; PMCID: PMC7035304.

66. A 72-year-old female is enrolled in a clinical trial evaluating a novel oral tyrosine kinase inhibitor for the treatment of advanced thyroid cancer. Pre-clinical studies suggested a possible impact on cardiac repolarization. Which of the following statements is correct regarding QT interval evaluation in patients undergoing cancer treatment?

A. QT interval prolongation is a more significant issue with arsenic trioxide than with nilotinib.

B. QT interval prolongation is rarely associated with oral cancer therapies.

C. The Bazett formula is the preferred correction formula for oncology patients.

D. Ventricular arrhythmias occur in greater than 10% of individuals with significant QT interval prolongation.

QTc prolongation in the context of arsenic trioxide therapy (e.g, while treating acute promyelocytic leukemia) can occur in up to 38% of patients. The risk with nilotinib therapy is less with QTc prolongation occurring in up to 24% of patients.

Reference(s):

- Porta-Sánchez A, Gilbert C, Spears D, Amir E, Chan J, Nanthakumar K, Thavendiranathan P. Incidence, Diagnosis, and Management of QT Prolongation Induced by Cancer Therapies: A Systematic Review. J Am Heart Assoc. 2017 Dec 7;6(12):e007724. doi: 10.1161/JAHA.117.007724. PMID: 29217664; PMCID: PMC5779062.

67. A 46-year-old female presents to clinic complaining of dyspnea on exertion and new lower extremity edema. She has gained 15 pounds (6.8 kilograms) over the past 3 weeks. Physical examination revealed an elevated jugular venous pressure, ascites, and 2+ bilateral lower extremity pitting edema. A limited, point-of-care echocardiogram showed a normal left ventricular systolic function. Her medical history includes prior Hodgkin lymphoma at the age of 14 years and treatment with mantle radiation. Which of the following test would be most helpful in establishing a diagnosis?

    A. Cardiac magnetic resonance imaging (CMR)

    B. Contrast-enhanced echocardiography

    C. Nuclear multigated acquisition scan (MUGA)

    D. Transesophageal echocardiogram

    The patient has most likely developed constrictive pericarditis due to prior radiation therapy to the chest as part of the treatment for Hodgkin lymphoma. In general, the first non-invasive test to evaluate for constrictive pericarditis is a transthoracic echocardiogram. When echocardiography cannot be used to establish a definitive diagnosis or when additional evaluation of the pericardium or tissue characterization (e.g., myocardial fibrosis) is warranted, CT or MRI can provide further information. Cardiac MRI with late gadolinium enhancement can provide information about ongoing pericardial inflammation. Moreover, cardiac MRI can also evaluate for ventricular interdependence with respiratory variation as well as determine blood flow velocities from atrioventricular valves and differential ventricular filling with respiration. A cardiac CT may provide useful information about pericardial anatomy, especially in patients being considered for pericardiectomy. It is also highly sensitive for detecting pericardial calcification.

    Chronic pericarditis may develop years after radiotherapy. Its prevalence has been estimated to be 7% to 20% in patients who received high-dose mantle radiotherapy for Hodgkin lymphoma. In addition to pericardial disease, patients who received mantle radiation are also at risk for developing myocardial fibrosis.

Reference(s):

- Groarke JD, Nguyen PL, Nohria A, Ferrari R, Cheng S, Moslehi J. Cardiovascular complications of radiation therapy for thoracic malignancies: the role for non-invasive imaging for detection of cardiovascular disease. Eur Heart J. 2014 Mar;35(10):612-23. doi: 10.1093/eurheartj/eht114. Epub 2013 May 10. PMID: 23666251; PMCID: PMC3945797.
- Mitchell JD, Cehic DA, Morgia M, Bergom C, Toohey J, Guerrero PA, Ferencik M, Kikuchi R, Carver JR, Zaha VG, Alvarez-Cardona JA, Szmit S, Daniele

AJ, Lopez-Mattei J, Zhang L, Herrmann J, Nohria A, Lenihan DJ, Dent SF. Cardiovascular Manifestations From Therapeutic Radiation: A Multidisciplinary Expert Consensus Statement From the International Cardio-Oncology Society. JACC CardioOncol. 2021 Sep 21;3(3):360-380. doi: 10.1016/j.jaccao.2021.06.003. PMID: 34604797; PMCID: PMC8463721.

- Syed FF, Schaff HV, Oh JK. Constrictive pericarditis--a curable diastolic heart failure. Nat Rev Cardiol. 2014 Sep;11(9):530-44. doi: 10.1038/nrcardio.2014.100. Epub 2014 Jul 29. Erratum in: Nat Rev Cardiol. 2015 Dec;12(12):682. PMID: 25072910.

68. A 56-year-old male with history of essential hypertension and mixed hyperlipidemia is about to start an anthracycline-based chemotherapy regimen. Which of the following imaging modalities is the most appropriate initial choice for assessing left ventricular function?

    A. Cardiac magnetic resonance imaging (MRI)

    B. Echocardiogram with strain imaging

    C. Nuclear multi-gated acquisition scan (MUGA)

    D. Nuclear stress test

    Echocardiography is the best initial modality to assess left ventricular function in patients starting anthracycline therapy. A comprehensive assessment with 3D volumetric and strain measurements allows more confident detection of clinical and subclinical cardiotoxicity on subsequent surveillance imaging.

Reference(s):

- Dobson R, Ghosh AK, Ky B, Marwick T, Stout M, Harkness A, Steeds R, Robinson S, Oxborough D, Adlam D, Stanway S, Rana B, Ingram T, Ring L, Rosen S, Plummer C, Manisty C, Harbinson M, Sharma V, Pearce K, Lyon AR, Augustine DX; British Society of Echocardiography (BSE) and the British Society of Cardio-Oncology (BCOS). BSE and BCOS Guideline for Transthoracic Echocardiographic Assessment of Adult Cancer Patients Receiving Anthracyclines and/or Trastuzumab. JACC CardioOncol. 2021 Mar 16;3(1):1-16. doi: 10.1016/j.jaccao.2021.01.011. PMID: 34396303; PMCID: PMC8352267.

69. Which of the following statements is correct about patients undergoing hematopoietic stem cell transplantation (HSCT)?

    A. Cyclophosphamide can cause significant cardiac morbidity in the acute setting

    B. HSCT is associated with a high prevalence of cardiac mortality

    C. HSCT is rarely associated with volume overload

    D. Late cardiotoxicity from cyclophosphamide is related to cumulative dose

    Cyclophosphamide-containing regimens can cause cardiotoxicity in 7-28% of patients. Most commonly this is seen within the first 1-3 weeks of starting therapy.

    A recent single-center retrospective cohort study including all consecutive patients who underwent allogeneic HSCT for hematologic malignant disease from January 2013 to June 2018 showed a cumulative incidence of early cardiac events of 19% in the post-transplant cyclophosphamide group and 6%e no-post-transplant cyclophosphamide group (p <0.001). The main early cardiac events after pos-transplant cyclophosphamide were left ventricular systolic dysfunction (13%), acute pulmonary edema (7%), pericarditis (4%), arrhythmia (3%), and acute coronary syndrome (2%). In multivariable analysis, the use of post-transplant cyclophosphamide was associated early cardiac events (hazard ratio, 2.7; 95% confidence interval, 1.4 to 4.9; p = 0.002).

Reference(s):

- Dhesi S, Chu MP, Blevins G, Paterson I, Larratt L, Oudit GY, Kim DH. Cyclophosphamide-Induced Cardiomyopathy: A Case Report, Review, and Recommendations for Management. J Investig Med High Impact Case Rep. 2013 Jan 1;1(1):2324709613480346. doi: 10.1177/2324709613480346. PMID: 26425570; PMCID: PMC4528786.
- Duléry R, Mohty R, Labopin M, Sestili S, Malard F, Brissot E, Battipaglia G, Médiavilla C, Banet A, Van de Wyngaert Z, Paviglianiti A, Belhocine R, Isnard F, Lapusan S, Adaeva R, Vekhoff A, Ledraa T, Legrand O, Cohen A, Bonnin A, Ederhy S, Mohty M. Early Cardiac Toxicity Associated With Post-Transplant Cyclophosphamide in Allogeneic Stem Cell Transplantation. JACC CardioOncol. 2021 Jun 15;3(2):250-259. doi: 10.1016/j.jaccao.2021.02.011. PMID: 34396331; PMCID: PMC8352028.

70. A 55-year-old male with multivessel coronary artery disease and severe mitral regurgitation will be undergoing coronary bypass grafting and mitral valve repair. He has been on bevacizumab and FOLFOX (folinic acid, 5-fluorouracil, and oxaliplatin) for 3 months for colon cancer. What would be a reason to delay surgery?

    A. Impaired platelet function

    B. Poor wound healing

    C. Recurrent ischemia with anesthesia

    D. Risk of hypertensive crisis

    Angiogenesis is crucial for wound healing. Bevacizumab being a vascular endothelial growth factor inhibitor is associated with an increased risk of impaired wound healing. Surgical patients on bevacizumab need close postoperative wound monitoring.

Reference(s):

- Scappaticci FA, Fehrenbacher L, Cartwright T, Hainsworth JD, Heim W, Berlin J, Kabbinavar F, Novotny W, Sarkar S, Hurwitz H. Surgical wound healing complications in metastatic colorectal cancer patients treated with bevacizumab. J Surg Oncol. 2005 Sep 1;91(3):173-80. doi: 10.1002/jso.20301. PMID: 16118771.
- Sharma K, Marcus JR. Bevacizumab and wound-healing complications: mechanisms of action, clinical evidence, and management recommendations for the plastic surgeon. Ann Plast Surg. 2013 Oct;71(4):434-40. doi: 10.1097/SAP.0b013e31824e5e57. PMID: 22868316.

71. A 55-year-old male presents with acute dyspnea and hypertensive urgency (186/122 mmHg). Blood pressure upon standing was 110/70 mmHg. What test would most likely be diagnostic?

A. Serum free light chains

B. Renal ultrasound

C. Serum catecholamines

D. Urine 5 HIAA

Adrenal tumors can cause hypertension with swinging blood pressure changes, headaches, hypokalemia and sweating. A good first screen is to measure serum catecholamines.

Previous studies have described orthostatic hypotension among patients with pheochromocytoma. Streeten and Anderson previously reported orthostatic hypotension and tachycardia to be present in 83% and 61%, respectively of 18 patients with subsequently proven pheochromocytoma.

Reference(s):

- Bhargava P, Sangster G, Haque K, Garrett J, Donato M, D'Agostino H. A Multimodality Review of Adrenal Tumors. CurrProblDiagnRadiol. 2019 Nov-Dec;48(6):605-615. doi: 10.1067/j.cpradiol.2018.10.002. Epub 2018 Oct 25. PMID: 30472137.
- Streeten DH, Anderson GH Jr. Mechanisms of orthostatic hypotension and tachycardia in patients with pheochromocytoma. Am J Hypertens. 1996 Aug;9(8):760-9. doi: 10.1016/0895-7061(96)00057-x. PMID: 8862222.

72. A 26-year-old female is seen by her obstetrician for a second trimester visit. A mass is discovered in her right breast and biopsy shows inflammatory breast cancer. Which of the following is a true statement regarding breast cancer and pregnancy?

A. Chemotherapy increases the risk of early delivery

B. Chemotherapy is safe during all trimesters

C. Pregnancy should be terminated

D. Breast surgery is her only option

In an international cohort study run by the International Network on Cancer, Infertility, and Pregnancy (INCIP) network, 61% of children prenatally exposed to chemotherapy were born pre-term (gestational age <37 weeks). Chemotherapy during pregnancy can also increase the risk of small for gestational age babies with an incidence of 7-17% depending on cancer type and chemotherapy administered.

Reference(s):

- Amant F, Vandenbroucke T, Verheecke M, Fumagalli M, Halaska MJ, Boere I, Han S, Gziri MM, Peccatori F, Rob L, Lok C, Witteveen P, Voigt JU, Naulaers G, Vallaeys L, Van den Heuvel F, Lagae L, Mertens L, Claes L, Van Calsteren K; International Network on Cancer, Infertility, and Pregnancy (INCIP). Pediatric

Outcome after Maternal Cancer Diagnosed during Pregnancy. N Engl J Med. 2015 Nov 5;373(19):1824-34. doi: 10.1056/NEJMoa1508913. Epub 2015 Sep 28. PMID: 26415085.

- Cardonick E, Iacobucci A. Use of chemotherapy during human pregnancy. Lancet Oncol. 2004 May;5(5):283-91. doi: 10.1016/S1470-2045(04)01466-4. PMID: 15120665.
- Chang A, Patel S. Treatment of acute myeloid leukemia during pregnancy. Ann Pharmacother. 2015 Jan;49(1):48-68. doi: 10.1177/1060028014552516. Epub 2014 Sep 25. PMID: 25258419.
- Luttwak E, Gurevich-Shapiro A, Azem F, Lishner M, Klieger C, Herishanu Y, Perry C, Avivi I. Novel agents for the treatment of lymphomas during pregnancy: A comprehensive literature review. Blood Rev. 2021 Sep;49:100831. doi: 10.1016/j.blre.2021.100831. Epub 2021 Apr 16. PMID: 33931297.

73. A 45-year-old male with acute myelogenous leukemia (AML) achieves remission after 7+3 induction (cytarabine and idarubicin) followed by allogeneic stem cell transplantation. He complains of almost disabling positional lightheadedness. On exam, supine blood pressure is 100/74 mmHg and standing blood pressure is 68/44 mmHg. Serum electrolytes are within normal range. What is the most likely cause of his orthostatic hypotension?

    A. Adrenal insufficiency
    B. Anthracycline cardiac toxicity
    C. Cytarabine cardiac toxicity
    D. Immune-mediated autonomic dysfunction

Reference(s):

- Mangaonkar A, Khateeb HA, Duma N, St Louis EK, McKeon A, Patnaik M, Hogan W, Litzow M, Kourelis T. Immune-Mediated Autonomic Neuropathies following Allogeneic Stem Cell Transplantation in Acute Myeloid Leukemia. Case Rep Hematol. 2017;2017:6803804. doi: 10.1155/2017/6803804. Epub 2017 Aug 27. PMID: 28928996; PMCID: PMC5591963.

74. Which of the following favors that a cardiac mass is malignant on a cardiac MRI?

    A. Abnormal first pass perfusion
    B. Left atrial location
    C. Narrow base of attachment
    D. Size 2-3 cm

    Abnormal first pass perfusion indicates that the mass has a vascular supply and thus more likely to be malignant. The other features described are in keeping with benign masses.

Reference(s):

- Tyebally S, Chen D, Bhattacharyya S, Mughrabi A, Hussain Z, Manisty C, Westwood M, Ghosh AK, Guha A. Cardiac Tumors: JACC CardioOncology State-of-the-Art Review. JACC CardioOncol. 2020 Jun 16;2(2):293-311. doi: 10.1016/j.jaccao.2020.05.009. PMID: 34396236; PMCID: PMC8352246.

75. Which of the following is true of imaging cardiac tumors?

   A. 3D echocardiography is superior to 2D echocardiography in assessing size
   B. A high carbohydrate diet is required to adequately evaluate cardiac tumors by FDG PET
   C. Microscopic calcification is best determined by cardiac MRI
   D. Use of ultrasound enhancing agent is FDA-approved to evaluate tumor perfusion

   3-dimensional (3D) echocardiography allows more accurate geometric assumptions to be made with volumetric imaging. Compared to 2-dimensional (2D) echocardiography more reproducible measurements are obtained and the full extent of cardiac masses can be seen.

Reference(s):

- Mankad R, Herrmann J. Cardiac tumors: echo assessment. Echo Res Pract. 2016 Dec;3(4):R65-R77. doi: 10.1530/ERP-16-0035. Epub 2016 Sep 6. PMID: 27600455; PMCID: PMC5292983.
- Tyebally S, Chen D, Bhattacharyya S, Mughrabi A, Hussain Z, Manisty C, Westwood M, Ghosh AK, Guha A. Cardiac Tumors: JACC CardioOncology State-of-the-Art Review. JACC CardioOncol. 2020 Jun 16;2(2):293-311. doi: 10.1016/j.jaccao.2020.05.009. PMID: 34396236; PMCID: PMC8352246.

76. In which clinical condition is cardiac MRI preferred over echocardiography?

   A. 5-fluorouracil associated acute coronary syndrome
   B. Cardiac tamponade
   C. Radiation-induced valvular heart disease
   D. Suspected myocarditis

   Myocarditis is a disease of the myocardium. Cardiac magnetic resonance (CMR) is the best modality for tissue characterization. CMR can help determine if there is localized or diffuse myocardial fibrosis in a case of suspected myocarditis and can also detect myocardial edema associated with myocardial inflammation.

Reference(s):

- Zhang L, Awadalla M, Mahmood SS, Nohria A, Hassan MZO, Thuny F, Zlotoff DA, Murphy SP, Stone JR, Golden DLA, Alvi RM, Rokicki A, Jones-O'Connor M, Cohen JV, Heinzerling LM, Mulligan C, Armanious M, Barac A, Forrestal BJ, Sullivan RJ, Kwong RY, Yang EH, Damrongwatanasuk R, Chen CL, Gupta D, Kirchberger MC, Moslehi JJ, Coelho-Filho OR, Ganatra S, Rizvi MA, Sahni G, Tocchetti CG, Mercurio V, Mahmoudi M, Lawrence DP, Reynolds KL, Weinsaft JW, Baksi AJ, Ederhy S, Groarke JD, Lyon AR, Fradley MG, Thavendiranathan P, Neilan TG. Cardiovascular magnetic resonance in immune checkpoint inhibitor-associated myocarditis. Eur Heart J. 2020 May 7;41(18):1733-1743. doi: 10.1093/eurheartj/ehaa051. PMID: 32112560; PMCID: PMC7205467.

77. A 62-year-old male with acute myeloid leukemia (AML) achieves remission after induction with 7+3 (cytarabine and idarubicin) and consolidation with HiDAC (high dose cytarabine). He undergoes a 10/10 matched unrelated donor allogeneic stem cell transplantation. His serum creatinine is 0.9 mg/dL, potassium 3.4 mmol/L, and magnesium 1.2 mg/dL. On day 12 post-stem cell transplant, he has the following electrocardiogram (ECG). Which of the following medications may contribute to this ECG abnormality?

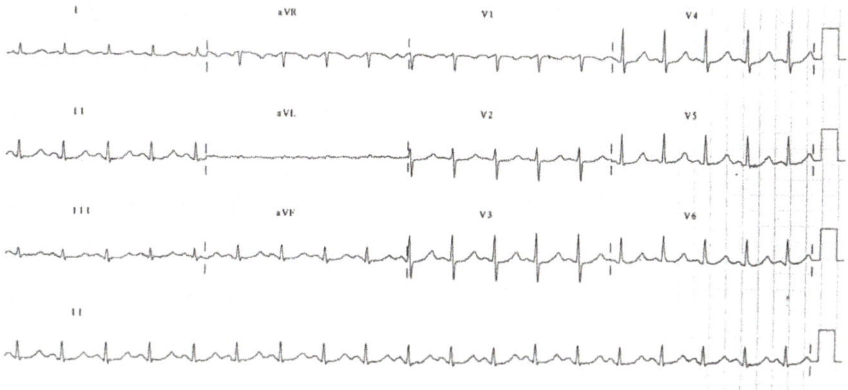

A. Acyclovir
B. Letermovir
C. Prednisone
D. Tacrolimus

Tacrolimus can cause QT interval prolongation, presumably as a result of tacrolimus-associated hypomagnesemia. Baseline and repeat electrocardiography should be carried out to assess for this with appropriate intervention depending upon the degree of prolongation. This is in addition to monitor closely for electrolyte abnormalities, such as hypomagnesemia, hypokalemia, and hypocalcemia.

Reference(s):

- Aisa Y, Mori T, Nakazato T, Shimizu T, Yamazaki R, Ikeda Y, Okamoto S. Effects of immunosuppressive agents on magnesium metabolism early after allogeneic hematopoietic stem cell transplantation. Transplantation. 2005 Oct 27;80(8):1046-50. doi: 10.1097/01.tp.0000174340.40585.d4. PMID: 16278584.
- Khatib R, Sabir FRN, Omari C, Pepper C, Tayebjee MH. Managing drug-induced QT prolongation in clinical practice. Postgrad Med J. 2021 Jul;97(1149):452-458. doi: 10.1136/postgradmedj-2020-138661. Epub 2020 Oct 29. PMID: 33122341; PMCID: PMC8237186.
- Navaneethan SD, Sankarasubbaiyan S, Gross MD, Jeevanantham V, Monk RD. Tacrolimus-associated hypomagnesemia in renal transplant recipients. Transplant Proc. 2006 Jun;38(5):1320-2. doi: 10.1016/j.transproceed.2006.02.077. PMID: 16797291.

78. A 47-year-old female is diagnosed with stage IV non-Hodgkin lymphoma with a high tumor burden. On day 5 of her treatment, she complains of nausea, vomiting, and palpitations. The nurse notices that her urine is "dark". Which of the following would you expect to see in checking her electrolytes?

A. Hypercalcemia
B. Hyperphosphatemia
C. Hypokalemia
D. Hypouricemia

Tumor lysis syndrome may result in hyperuricemia, hyperkalemia, hyperphosphatemia, and hypocalcemia. It is more common in high tumor burden states treated with chemotherapy and is regarded as an oncometabolic emergency resulting from rapid cell death.

Reference(s):

- Mirrakhimov AE, Voore P, Khan M, Ali AM. Tumor lysis syndrome: A clinical review. World J Crit Care Med. 2015 May 4;4(2):130-8. doi: 10.5492/wjccm.v4.i2.130. PMID: 25938028; PMCID: PMC4411564.

79. A 49-year-old female who is 11 months post renal transplant presents with new onset of fever and dyspnea. She has a bulky mediastinal mass on chest imaging. A biopsy of the mass is consistent with CD20+ post-transplant lymphoproliferative disease (PTLD). What is the most effective treatment for her?

A. Allogeneic stem cell transplantation
B. Everolimus
C. Mediastinal radiation
D. Rituximab

Rituxumab is an effective treatment for PTLD. In patients who have an inadequate response to reduction of immunosuppression, the humanized anti-CD20 monoclonal antibody rituximab has become a standard of care. Rituximab can be given as monotherapy or in combination with chemotherapy, concurrently or sequentially. Reports have demonstrated the safety and efficacy of single-agent rituximab in the treatment of CD20-expressing PTLD, generally with a response rate of approximately 50%.

Reference(s):

- Gordan LN, Grow WB, Pusateri A, Douglas V, Mendenhall NP, Lynch JW. Phase II trial of individualized rituximab dosing for patients with CD20-positive lymphoproliferative disorders. J Clin Oncol. 2005 Feb 20;23(6):1096-102. doi: 10.1200/JCO.2005.12.171. Epub 2005 Jan 18. PMID: 15657402.
- Samant H, Vaitla P, Kothadia JP. Post Transplant Lymphoproliferative Disorders. 2022 Jul 12. In: StatPearls [Internet]. Treasure Island (FL): StatPearls Publishing; 2022 Jan–. PMID: 30020621.

80. A 23-year-old male with sickle cell disease is admitted with a vaso-occlusive crisis and anemia. On exam, his temperature is 99° Fahrenheit (37.2° Celsius), blood pressure is 124/75 mmHg, and pulse is 110 beats per minute. His oxygen saturation on room air is 98%. He is transfused 2 units of packed red blood cells (PRBCs) for worsening anemia. At the end of his second unit of PRBCs, he reports shortness of breath. Physical examination reveals diffuse bilateral crackles, jugular venous distention, and an S3 on cardiac auscultation. A chest X-ray shows diffuse bilateral infiltrates. What is the most likely diagnosis?

A. Acute chest syndrome

B. Acute pulmonary embolism

C. Transfusion associated circulatory overload (TACO)

D. Transfusion related acute lung injury (TRALI)

TACO is an established, but grossly under diagnosed and underreported complication of blood transfusion. Identifying its presence and distinguishing it from transfusion-related acute lung injury (TRALI) is key to selecting appropriate management and treatment options. Though similar to TACO, TRALI has a few distinguishing characteristics, such as hypotension versus hypertension, lack of widened pulse pressure, exudate pulmonary edema fluid, balanced fluids, and minimal response to diuretics.

Reference(s):

- Agnihotri N, Agnihotri A. Transfusion associated circulatory overload. Indian J Crit Care Med. 2014 Jun;18(6):396-8. doi: 10.4103/0972-5229.133938. PMID: 24987240; PMCID: PMC4071685.
- Arzoun H, Srinivasan M, Adam M, Thomas SS, Lee B, Yarema A. A Systematic Review on the Management of Transfusion-Related Acute Lung Injury in Transfusion-Dependent Sickle Cell Disease. Cureus. 2022 Feb 10;14(2):e22101. doi: 10.7759/cureus.22101. PMID: 35165647; PMCID: PMC8830742.

81. Which of the following statements is true regarding patients with thalassemia?

A. Cardiac iron overload with heart failure can be successfully reversed with early, aggressive chelation therapy.

B. Cardiovascular complications are rarely a cause of death in transfusion-dependent thalassemia patients.

C. Routine screening for iron overload with cardiac magnetic imaging is now recommended

D. Sildenafil has been shown to have no benefit in thalassemia patients who develop pulmonary hypertension.

There is no role for screening asymptomatic thalassemia patients with normal left ventricular function for iron overload using cardiac magnetic resonance imaging. Therapeutic phlebotomy is the therapy of choice in nonanemic patients with cardiac hemochromatosis. Phlebotomy is not an option for therapy in patients with anemia (secondary iron-overload disorders) nor in patients with severe heart failure. In these patients, the therapy of choice is iron chelation treatment.

Iron chelating agents increase the iron excretion rate by binding to the iron in plasma and tissues, depleting the body of excess iron.

Reference(s):

- Fabio G, Minonzio F, Delbini P, Bianchi A, Cappellini MD. Reversal of cardiac complications by deferiprone and deferoxamine combination therapy in a patient affected by a severe type of juvenile hemochromatosis (JH). Blood. 2007 Jan 1;109(1):362-4. doi: 10.1182/blood-2006-04-016949. Epub 2006 Sep 7. PMID: 16960153.
- Glickstein H, El RB, Link G, Breuer W, Konijn AM, Hershko C, Nick H, Cabantchik ZI. Action of chelators in iron-loaded cardiac cells: Accessibility to intracellular labile iron and functional consequences. Blood. 2006 Nov 1;108(9):3195-203. doi: 10.1182/blood-2006-05-020867. Epub 2006 Jul 11. PMID: 16835377.
- Kontoghiorghes GJ, Eracleous E, Economides C, Kolnagou A. Advances in iron overload therapies. prospects for effective use of deferiprone (L1), deferoxamine, the new experimental chelators ICL670, GT56-252, L1NA11 and their combinations. Curr Med Chem. 2005;12(23):2663-81. doi: 10.2174/092986705774463003. PMID: 16305464.

82. A 70-year-old male with acute myeloid leukemia (ALL) is receiving treatment with venetoclax. He is currently on amlodipine, carvedilol, and lisinopril for essential hypertension and rosuvastatin for mixed hyperlipidemia. Which of his current medications has the potential for significant drug-drug interaction with his cancer therapy?

    A. Amlodipine

    B. Carvedilol

    C. Lisinopril

    D. Rosuvastatin

    Concomitant use of venetoclax with a strong or moderate CYP3A inhibitor or P-gp inhibitor increases the concentration of venetoclax, which may in turn increase its toxicities, including the risk of tumor lysis syndrome. In patients with chronic lymphocytic leukemia/small lymphocytic lymphoma, concomitant use with a strong CYP3A inhibitor at initiation and during the ramp-up phase is contraindicated. If concomitant use with a P-gp inhibitor is not possible, the recommendation is to separate dosing of the P-gp inhibitor (e.g., carvedilol) at least 6 hours before venetoclax.

Reference(s):

- AbbVie, Inc. Venclexta (venetoclax) [package insert]. U.S. Food and Drug Administration website. https://www.accessdata.fda.gov/drugsatfda_docs/label/2016/208573s000lbl.pdf. Revised April 2016. Accessed November 28, 2022.

83. A 35-year-old male with history of Hodgkin lymphoma treated with radiation therapy and ABVD (doxorubicin, bleomycin, vincristine, and dacarbazine) 15 years ago would like to know if he has any sports restrictions. Which of the following sports could be associated with a higher risk of cardiopulmonary complications in this patient?

A. Baseball
B. Scuba diving
C. Soccer
D. Swimming

Approximately 10% of patients treated with bleomycin may experience a pulmonary adverse reaction. The most frequent presentation is pneumonitis, which occasionally progresses to pulmonary fibrosis. Pulmonary toxicity is both dose and age related, being more common in patients over the age of 70 years and in those receiving more than 400 units. In general, patients who have been treated with bleomycin are at greater risk of developing pulmonary toxicity when exposed to high concentrations of oxygen, such as during surgery or scuba diving.

Reference(s):

- Nippon Kayaku Co., Ltd., and Bristol-Myers Squibb Company. Blenoxane (bleomycin sulfate) [package insert]. U.S. Food and Drug Administration website. https://www.accessdata.fda.gov/drugsatfda_docs/label/2010/050443s036lbl.pdf. Revised April 2010. Accessed on November 30, 2022.
- Shippee BM, Bates JS, Richards KL. The role of screening and monitoring for bleomycin pulmonary toxicity. J Oncol Pharm Pract. 2016 Apr;22(2):308-12. doi: 10.1177/1078155215574294. Epub 2015 Mar 2. PMID: 25736276.
- van Hulst RA, Rietbroek RC, Gaastra MT, Schlösser NJ. To dive or not to dive with bleomycin: a practical algorithm. Aviat Space Environ Med. 2011 Aug;82(8):814-8. doi: 10.3357/asem.2816.2011. PMID: 21853861.
- Zorzi AP, Yang CL, Dell S, Nathan PC. Bleomycin-associated Lung Toxicity in Childhood Cancer Survivors. J PediatrHematol Oncol. 2015 Nov;37(8):e447-52. doi: 10.1097/MPH.0000000000000424. PMID: 26422284.
- Brandt JP, Gerriets V. Bleomycin. [Updated 2022 Aug 29]. In: StatPearls [Internet]. Treasure Island (FL): StatPearls Publishing; 2022 Jan-. Available from: https://www.ncbi.nlm.nih.gov/books/NBK555895/

84. What is the principal role of the cardio-oncologist during cancer treatment?

A. Apply target doses of evidence-based heart failure medications
B. Maintain left ventricular ejection fraction within normal range
C. Monitor imaging and blood markers of cardiotoxicity
D. Support safe continuation of cancer therapy

The cardiovascular care of the oncology patient is a collaborative effort among different healthcare providers (e.g., oncologist, hematologist, cardiologist, radiologist, surgeons, palliative care specialists, etc.). The cardio-oncologist's role is to support safe continuation of cancer therapy by preventing, diagnosing, and treating potential cardiovascular complications related to the cancer itself or its treatment.

Reference(s):

- Adusumalli S, Alvarez-Cardona J, Khatana SM, Mitchell JD, Blaes AH, Casselli SJ, O'Quinn R, Lenihan DJ. Clinical Practice and Research in Cardio-Oncology: Finding the "Rosetta Stone" for Establishing Program Excellence in Cardio-oncology. J Cardiovasc Transl Res. 2020 Jun;13(3):495-505. doi: 10.1007/s12265-020-10010-x. Epub 2020 May 22. PMID: 32444945.
- Ghosh AK, Walker JM. Cardio-Oncology - A new subspecialty with collaboration at its heart. Indian Heart J. 2017 Jul-Aug;69(4):556-562. doi: 10.1016/j.ihj.2017.05.006. Epub 2017 May 27. PMID: 28822531; PMCID: PMC5560887.
- Lenihan DJ, Mitchell J, Alvarez-Cardona J. A practical approach to the evaluation of a cardio-oncology patient. In: Lenihan DJ, Mitchell JD, Zhang KW, editors. The Washington Manual of Cardio-Oncology: A Practical Guide for Improved Cancer Survivorship. 1st ed. Wolters Kluwer; 2022. p. 1-25. ISBN: 9781975180447.

85. Which of the following statements best describes the long-term risk of cardiotoxicity from anthracyclines in childhood cancer survivors?

   A. Dexrazoxane reduces the risk of cardiotoxicity when administered before each dose of doxorubicin.

   B. Doxorubicin given by continuous infusion is no safer than bolus therapy.

   C. Mitoxantrone is associated with a lower risk of cardiotoxicity when compared to doxorubicin.

   D. Surveillance for cardiac dysfunction should be performed more frequently if treatment was given after puberty.

Dexrazoxane is an effective cardioprotectant when administered with anthracycline chemotherapy. It is not associated with a reduction in anti-tumor efficacy or survival nor is it associated with a relevant increased risk of second primary malignancies. As such it is recommended as a cardioprotectant particularly for children and adolescents for whom the development of anthracycline-induced cardiotoxicity could have a crucial prognostic impact.

Reference(s):

- Asselin BL, Devidas M, Chen L, Franco VI, Pullen J, Borowitz MJ, Hutchison RE, Ravindranath Y, Armenian SH, Camitta BM, Lipshultz SE. Cardioprotection and Safety of Dexrazoxane in Patients Treated for Newly Diagnosed T-Cell Acute Lymphoblastic Leukemia or Advanced-Stage Lymphoblastic Non-Hodgkin Lymphoma: A Report of the Children's Oncology Group Randomized Trial Pediatric Oncology Group 9404. J Clin Oncol. 2016 Mar 10;34(8):854-62. doi: 10.1200/JCO.2015.60.8851. Epub 2015 Dec 23. Erratum in: J Clin Oncol. 2017 Jun 20;35(18):2100. PMID: 26700126; PMCID: PMC4872007.
- Reichardt P, Tabone MD, Mora J, Morland B, Jones RL. Risk-benefit of dexrazoxane for preventing anthracycline-related cardiotoxicity: re-evaluating the European labeling. Future Oncol. 2018 Oct;14(25):2663-2676. doi: 10.2217/fon-2018-0210. Epub 2018 May 11. PMID: 29747541.

- van Dalen EC, Caron HN, Dickinson HO, Kremer LC. Cardioprotective interventions for cancer patients receiving anthracyclines. Cochrane Database Syst Rev. 2011 Jun 15;2011(6):CD003917. doi: 10.1002/14651858.CD003917.pub4. PMID: 21678342; PMCID: PMC6457676.

86. Which of the following tyrosine kinase inhibitor (TKI) causes significant hyperlipidemia?

    A. Alectinib

    B. Brigatinib

    C. Lorlatinib

    D. Ponatinib

    Lorlatinib is an oral, third-generation ALK/ROS1 tyrosine kinase inhibitor that is FDA-approved for the treatment of adult patients with metastatic non-small cell lung cancer whose tumors are anaplastic lymphoma kinase-positive. Its safety profile was established in a phase II clinical study. The most common adverse effects of any grade included hypercholesterolemia, hypertriglyceridemia, edema, peripheral neuropathy, weight gain, cognitive effects, mood effects, fatigue, diarrhea, arthralgia, and AST increased. The most commonly reported grade 4 adverse effects were hypercholesterolemia and hypertriglyceridemia. This is usually manageable with lipid-lowering therapy.

Reference(s):

- Bauer TM, Felip E, Solomon BJ, Thurm H, Peltz G, Chioda MD, Shaw AT. Clinical Management of Adverse Events Associated with Lorlatinib. Oncologist. 2019 Aug;24(8):1103-1110. doi: 10.1634/theoncologist.2018-0380. Epub 2019 Mar 19. PMID: 30890623; PMCID: PMC6693708.
- Solomon BJ, Besse B, Bauer TM, Felip E, Soo RA, Camidge DR, Chiari R, Bearz A, Lin CC, Gadgeel SM, Riely GJ, Tan EH, Seto T, James LP, Clancy JS, Abbattista A, Martini JF, Chen J, Peltz G, Thurm H, Ou SI, Shaw AT. Lorlatinib in patients with ALK-positive non-small-cell lung cancer: results from a global phase 2 study. Lancet Oncol. 2018 Dec;19(12):1654-1667. doi: 10.1016/S1470-2045(18)30649-1. Epub 2018 Nov 6. Erratum in: Lancet Oncol. 2019 Jan;20(1):e10. PMID: 30413378.

87. Certain cancer therapeutics can cause hypertriglyceridemia. Which of the following drugs is least likely to significantly elevate serum triglycerides?

    A. Anastrozole

    B. Asparaginase

    C. Brentuximab

    D. Capecitabine

    Out of all the above agents, only anastrozole is associated with a reduction in serum triglyceride levels. In the Tamoxifen Exemestane Adjuvant Multinational (TEAM) Japanese sub-study, a total of 154 breast cancer patients were assigned to receive exemestane, anastrozole, or tamoxifen. Triglycerides level among those who received anastrozole were not significantly affected. Asparaginase, brentuximab, and capecitabine have all been associated with hypertriglyceridemia.

Reference(s):

- Hozumi Y, Suemasu K, Takei H, Aihara T, Takehara M, Saito T, Ohsumi S, Masuda N, Ohashi Y. The effect of exemestane, anastrozole, and tamoxifen on lipid profiles in Japanese postmenopausal early breast cancer patients: final results of National Surgical Adjuvant Study BC 04, the TEAM Japan sub-study. Ann Oncol. 2011 Aug;22(8):1777-82. doi: 10.1093/annonc/mdq707. Epub 2011 Feb 1. PMID: 21285133.
- Lu HH, Li Q, Xu BH, Zhang P, Yuan P, Wang JY, Cai RG. [Effects of anastrozole on lipid metabolism in Chinese postmenopausal women with breast cancer]. Zhonghua Zhong Liu Za Zhi. 2011 Jul;33(7):520-5. Chinese. PMID: 22093630.
- Sawada S, Sato K, Kusuhara M, Ayaori M, Yonemura A, Tamaki K, Hiraide H, Mochizuki H, Ohsuzu F. Effect of anastrozole and tamoxifen on lipid metabolism in Japanese postmenopausal women with early breast cancer. Acta Oncol. 2005;44(2):134-41. doi: 10.1080/02841860510007585. PMID: 15788292.

88. Which of the following is the most accurate statement regarding radiation therapy for breast cancer?

    A. Deep-inspiration breath holding (DIBH) during treatment minimizes cardiac exposure
    B. Doubling the number of radiation fractions reduces the risk of toxicity
    C. One single high dose treatment is effective treatment and eliminates cardiac toxicity
    D. There is no difference in late cardiac toxicity between left and right sided breast cancer treatment

The DIBH technique involves the patient inspiring to a specified threshold and then holding that level of inspiration during every radiation therapy field delivered. The use of this technique can be associated with lower radiation exposure to the heart without compromising coverage of the breast or chest wall. A number of studies have shown a reduction in the mean heart dose.

Reference(s):

- Bergom C, Currey A, Desai N, Tai A, Strauss JB. Deep Inspiration Breath Hold: Techniques and Advantages for Cardiac Sparing During Breast Cancer Irradiation. Front Oncol. 2018 Apr 4;8:87. doi: 10.3389/fonc.2018.00087. PMID: 29670854; PMCID: PMC5893752.
- Borst GR, Sonke JJ, den Hollander S, Betgen A, Remeijer P, van Giersbergen A, Russell NS, Elkhuizen PH, Bartelink H, van Vliet-Vroegindeweij C. Clinical results of image-guided deep inspiration breath hold breast irradiation. Int J Radiat Oncol Biol Phys. 2010 Dec 1;78(5):1345-51. doi: 10.1016/j.ijrobp.2009.10.006. Epub 2010 Mar 6. PMID: 20207496.

- Hayden AJ, Rains M, Tiver K. Deep inspiration breath hold technique reduces heart dose from radiotherapy for left-sided breast cancer. J Med Imaging Radiat Oncol. 2012 Aug;56(4):464-72. doi: 10.1111/j.1754-9485.2012.02405.x. PMID: 22883657.
- McIntosh A, Shoushtari AN, Benedict SH, Read PW, Wijesooriya K. Quantifying the reproducibility of heart position during treatment and corresponding delivered heart dose in voluntary deep inhalation breath hold for left breast cancer patients treated with external beam radiotherapy. Int J Radiat Oncol Biol Phys. 2011 Nov 15;81(4):e569-76. doi: 10.1016/j.ijrobp.2011.01.044. Epub 2011 Apr 29. PMID: 21531087.
- Mitchell JD, Cehic DA, Morgia M, Bergom C, Toohey J, Guerrero PA, Ferencik M, Kikuchi R, Carver JR, Zaha VG, Alvarez-Cardona JA, Szmit S, Daniele AJ, Lopez-Mattei J, Zhang L, Herrmann J, Nohria A, Lenihan DJ, Dent SF. Cardiovascular Manifestations From Therapeutic Radiation: A Multidisciplinary Expert Consensus Statement From the International Cardio-Oncology Society. JACC CardioOncol. 2021 Sep 21;3(3):360-380. doi: 10.1016/j.jaccao.2021.06.003. PMID: 34604797; PMCID: PMC8463721.
- Stranzl H, Zurl B. Postoperative irradiation of left-sided breast cancer patients and cardiac toxicity. Does deep inspiration breath-hold (DIBH) technique protect the heart? StrahlentherOnkol. 2008 Jul;184(7):354-8. doi: 10.1007/s00066-008-1852-0. Epub 2008 Oct 1. PMID: 19016033.

89. Which of the following is correct about anthracycline-associated cardiac toxicity?

    A. If there is no overt cardiac toxicity at 10 years after treatment completion, there is no further risk

    B. The risk of cardiac toxicity is less with hematologic compared to solid malignancies

    C. Topoisomerase 2-ß has been implicated

    D. Toxicity never occurs when the cumulative dose is less than 100 mg/m^2

    The basic mechanisms of anthracycline cardiotoxicity may involve direct pathways for reactive oxygen species generation and topoisomerase 2 as well as other indirect pathways. Late effects can occur decades after completion of anthracycline therapy. Cardiotoxicity is more common with hematological malignancies and can occur with any dose of anthracycline (although more likely with higher doses).

Reference(s):

- Cardinale D, Iacopo F, Cipolla CM. Cardiotoxicity of Anthracyclines. Front Cardiovasc Med. 2020 Mar 18;7:26. doi: 10.3389/fcvm.2020.00026. PMID: 32258060; PMCID: PMC7093379.
- McGowan JV, Chung R, Maulik A, Piotrowska I, Walker JM, Yellon DM. Anthracycline Chemotherapy and Cardiotoxicity. Cardiovasc Drugs Ther. 2017 Feb;31(1):63-75. doi: 10.1007/s10557-016-6711-0. PMID: 28185035; PMCID: PMC5346598

90. A 48-year-old female with history of Hodgkin lymphoma at the age of 17 years was treated with mantle radiation. She was recently diagnosed with metastatic ovarian carcinoma and has received one cycle of gemcitabine and cisplatin. She complains of pleuritic anterior chest pain and has a pericardial friction rub on exam. What is the most likely cause of her symptoms?

A. Acute pulmonary embolism

B. Coronary artery spasm

C. Metastatic disease to the lungs

D. Radiation recall

Radiation recall refers to an acute inflammatory reaction involving a previously irradiated area, and it is triggered by the administration of precipitating systemic agents after radiation treatment. The most common agents associated with this phenomenon are anticancer agents (bevacizumab plus gemcitabine, capecitabine, cyclophosphamide, docetaxel, doxorubicin, among others), but other drugs such as some antibiotics, antituberculosis drugs, and simvastatin have also been associated. Radiation recall can occur days, months or even years after irradiation. The pathophysiological mechanism of cutaneous radiation recall is not known, and various hypotheses have been postulated. Interestingly, many patients who develop radiation recall have no reaction to radiation during or at the end of radiotherapy. It most commonly presents on the skin, and it is usually mild to moderate in severity.

Reference(s):

- Burris HA 3rd, Hurtig J. Radiation recall with anticancer agents. Oncologist. 2010;15(11):1227-37. doi: 10.1634/theoncologist.2009-0090. Epub 2010 Nov 2. PMID: 21045191; PMCID: PMC3227903.

91. Which of the following is a contraindication to radiation therapy in breast cancer?

A. Active scleroderma with vasculitis

B. Diffusing capacity of the lungs for carbon monoxide (DLCO) 90% of the predicted value

C. Presence of a cardiac pacemaker

D. Prior localized radiation therapy for endometrial carcinoma

The decision to offer radiotherapy in patients with connective tissue diseases continues to be challenging.

Radiotherapy might trigger the onset of connective tissue diseases by increasing the expression of self-antigens, diminishing regulatory T-cell activity, and activating effectors of innate immunity (dendritic cells) through Toll-like receptor-dependent mechanisms, all of which could potentially lead to breaks of immune tolerance. Although generally well tolerated, radiation therapy in the setting of collagen vascular disease appears to carry a higher risk of late toxicity.

Reference(s):

- Shah DJ, Hirpara R, Poelman CL, Woods A, Hummers LK, Wigley FM, Wright JL, Parekh A, Steen VD, Domsic RT, Shah AA. Impact of Radiation Therapy on Scleroderma and Cancer Outcomes in Scleroderma Patients With Breast Cancer. Arthritis Care Res (Hoboken). 2018 Oct;70(10):1517-1524. doi: 10.1002/acr.23505. PMID: 29316366; PMCID: PMC6033679.
- Yoon SM, Chu FI, Ruan D, Steinberg ML, Raldow A, Lee P. Assessment of Toxic Effects Associated With Dose-Fractionated Radiotherapy Among Patients With Cancer and Comorbid Collagen Vascular Disease. JAMA Netw Open. 2021 Feb 1;4(2):e2034074. doi: 10.1001/jamanetworkopen.2020.34074. PMID: 33599771; PMCID: PMC7893499.

92. Which of the following drugs is a cyclin-dependent kinase (CDK) 4/6 inhibitor associated with QT interval prolongation?

    A. Nilotinib

    B. Palbociclib

    C. Ribociclib

    D. Temozolomide

    Nilotinib is a kinase inhibitor approved by the U.S. Food and Drug Administration (FDA) for the treatment of newly diagnosed adult patients with Philadelphia chromosome positive chronic myeloid leukemia (Ph+ CML) in chronic phase, and for the treatment of chronic phase and accelerated phase Ph+ CML in adult patients resitant to or intolerant to prior therapy that included imatinib. It is contraindicated in patients with hypokalemia, hypomagnesemia, or long QT syndrome. The FDA recommends obtaining an electrocardiogram (ECG) at baseline, 7 days after initiation, and periodically thereafter, and following any dose adjustments. The FDA also recommends avoiding use of concomitant drugs known to prolong the QT interval and strong CYP3A inhibitors.

    Temozolomide is an alkylating drug approved by the U.S. FDA for the treatment of adult patients with newly diagnosed glioblastoma multiforme concomitantly with radiotherapy and then as maintenance treatment, and for the treatment of refractory anaplastic astrocytoma in patients who have experienced disease progression on a drug regimen containing nitrosourea and procarbazine. It is associated with myelosuppression, Pneumocystis pneumonia, hepatotoxicity, and fetal toxicity.

CDK 4/6 Inhibitor	Indication(s)	Adverse Reactions	Recommendations
Ribociclib (Kisqali®)	Hormone receptor positive, HER2-negative advanced or metastatic breast cancer in combination with (1) an aromatase inhibitor as initial endocrine-based therapy; or (2) fulvestrant as initial endocrine-based therapy or following disease progression on endocrine therapy in postmenopausal women or in men	▪ QT interval prolongation ▪ Interstitial lung disease or pneumonitis ▪ Severe cutaneous adverse reactions (Stevens-Johnson syndrome, toxic epidermal necrolysis, and drug-reaction with eosinophilia and systemic symptoms) ▪ Hepatobiliary toxicity ▪ Neutropenia ▪ Embryo-fetal toxicity	QT interval prolongation: ▪ Electrocardiogram (ECG) and eletrolytes prior to initiation ▪ Repeat ECG at approximately day 14 of the first cycle and at the beginning of the second cycle, then as clinically indicated ▪ Avoid concomitant use of drugs known to prolong QT interval ▪ Avoiding concomitant use with strong CYP3A inhibitors or inducers
Palbociclib (Ibrance®)	Hormone receptor-positive, HER2-negative advanced or metastatic breast cancer in combination with (1) an aromatase inhibitor as initial endocrine-based therapy in postmenopausal women or men; or (2) fulvestrant in patients with disease progression following endocrine therapy.	▪ Neutropenia ▪ Interstitial lung disease or pneumonitis ▪ Embryo-fetal toxicity	▪ Avoid concurrent use with strong CYP3A inhibitors or inducers

Abemaciclib (Verzenio®)	■ In combination with endocrine therapy (tamoxifen or an aromatase inhibitor) for the adjuvant treatment of hormone-receptor positive, HER-2 negative, node-positive, early breast cancer at high risk of recurrence and a Ki-67 score ~20% ■ In combination with an aromatase inhibitor as initial endocrine-based therapy for the treatment of postmenopausal women, and men, with hormone receptor-positive, HER2-negative advanced or metastatic breast cancer ■ In combination with fulvestrant for the treatment of adult patients with hormone receptor-positive, HER-2 negative advanced or metastatic breast cancer with disease progression following endocrine therapy ■ As monotherapy for hormone-receptor positive, HER-2 negative advanced or metastatic breast cancer with disease progression following endocrine therapy and prior chemotherapy in the metastatic setting	■ Diarrhea ■ Neutropenia ■ Interstitial lung disease or pneumonitis ■ Hepatotoxicity ■ Venous thromboembolism ■ Embryo-fetal toxicity	■ Avoid concomitant use of ketoconazole ■ Reduce dose with concomitant use of other strong and moderate CYP3A inhibitors ■ Avoid concomitant use of strong and moderate CYP3A inducers

Reference(s):

- Eli Lilly and Company. Verzenio (abemaciclib) [package insert]. U.S. Food and Drug Administration website. https://www.accessdata.fda.gov/drugsatfda_docs/label/2021/208716s006s007s008lbl.pdf. Revised October 2021. Accessed on November 30, 2022.
- Merck & Co., Inc. Temodar (temozolomide) [package insert]. U.S. Food and Drug Administration website. https://www.accessdata.fda.gov/drugsatfda_docs/label/2016/021029s031lbl.pdf. Revised September 2015. Accessed on November 30, 2022.
- Novartis Pharmaceuticals Corporation. Kisqali (ribociblib) [package insert]. U.S. Food and Drug Administration website. https://www.accessdata.fda.gov/drugsatfda_docs/label/2021/209092s009lbl.pdf. Revised September 2021. Accessed on November 30, 2022.
- Novartis Pharmaceuticals Corporation. Tasigna (nilotinib) [package insert]. U.S. Food and Drug Administration website. https://www.accessdata.fda.gov/drugsatfda_docs/label/2017/022068s026lbl.pdf. Revised December 2017. Accessed on November 30, 2022.
- Pfizer Labs. Ibrance (palbociclib) [package insert]. U.S. Food and Drug Administration website. https://www.accessdata.fda.gov/drugsatfda_docs/label/2019/207103s008lbl.pdf. Revised April 2019. Accessed on November 30, 2022.

93. A 68-year-old male being treated for mantle cell lymphoma complains of palpitations and lightheadedness. A 24-hour Holter monitor reveals a 15-beat run of monomorphic ventricular tachycardia. Which of the following cancer therapeutics is the most likely cause of his arrhythmia?

    A. Fludarabine

    B. Ibrutinib

    C. Rituximab

    D. Vincristine

    Ibrutinib is a Bruton tyrosine kinase inhibitor that is indicated for the treatment of adult patients with mantle cell lymphoma who have received at least one prior therapy, chronic lymphocytic leukemia (CLL)/small lymphocytic lymphoma (SLL) with or without 17p deletion, Waldenström's macroglobulinemia, marginal zone lymphoma who require systemic therapy and have received at least one prior anti-CD20-based therapy, and chronic graft versus host disease after failure of one or more lines of systemic therapy.

    Ibrutinib has been reported to cause polymorphic ventricular tachycardia (VT) without QT interval prolongation as well as in the absence of structural heart disease. In a disproportionality analysis based on adverse drug reactions reported within VigiBase, ibrutinib was found to be associated with higher reporting of supraventricular arrhythmias (reporting odds ratios [ROR]: 23.1; 95% confidence interval [CI]: 21.6 to 24.7; $p < 0.0001$) and ventricular arrhythmias (ROR: 4.7; 95% CI: 3.7 to 5.9; $p < 0.0001$). Other cardiovascular adverse effects reported from the use of ibrutinib include heart failure, conduction disorders, central nervous system hemorrhagic events, and hypertension.

Reference(s):

- Du B, Chakraborty P, Azam MA, Massé S, Lai PFH, Niri A, Si D, Thavendiranathan P, Abdel-Qadir H, Billia F, Nanthakumar K. Acute Effects of Ibrutinib on Ventricular Arrhythmia in Spontaneously Hypertensive Rats. JACC CardioOncol. 2020 Nov 17;2(4):614-629. doi: 10.1016/j.jaccao.2020.08.012. PMID: 34396273; PMCID: PMC8352013.
- Lampson BL, Yu L, Glynn RJ, Barrientos JC, Jacobsen ED, Banerji V, Jones JA, Walewska R, Savage KJ, Michaud GF, Moslehi JJ, Brown JR. Ventricular arrhythmias and sudden death in patients taking ibrutinib. Blood. 2017 May 4;129(18):2581-2584. doi: 10.1182/blood-2016-10-742437. Epub 2017 Feb 21. PMID: 28223277; PMCID: PMC7219062.
- Salem JE, Manouchehri A, Bretagne M, Lebrun-Vignes B, Groarke JD, Johnson DB, Yang T, Reddy NM, Funck-Brentano C, Brown JR, Roden DM, Moslehi JJ. Cardiovascular Toxicities Associated With Ibrutinib. J Am Coll Cardiol. 2019 Oct 1;74(13):1667-1678. doi: 10.1016/j.jacc.2019.07.056. PMID: 31558250.

94. A 45-year-old female with metastatic melanoma is started on combination therapy with dabrafenib and trametinib. Which of the following is the most likely cardiovascular complication with this therapy?

    A. Cardiomyopathy
    B. Pericardial effusion
    C. Pleural effusion
    D. QT interval prolongation

    The combination of dabrafenib and trametinib is indicated for the treatment of patients with unresectable or metastatic melanoma with BRAF V600E or V600K mutations, the adjuvant treatment of patients with melanoma with BRAF V600E or V600K mutations and involvement of lymph nodes following complete resection, treatment of patients with metastatic non-small cell lung cancer with BRAF V600E mutations, and treatment of patients with locally advanced or metastatic anaplastic thyroid cancer with BRAF V600E mutation and with no satisfactory locoregional treatment options.

    A pooled analysis of data from the intention-to-treat population of previously untreated patients who had metastatic melanoma with a BRAF V600E or V600K mutation in the COMBI-d trial and the COMBI-v trial showed that the most common adverse events that led to permanent discontinuation of treatment drugs were pyrexia in 23 patients (4%), decreased ejection fraction in 21 patients (4%), and an increased alanine aminotransferase level in 7 patients (1%). No deaths were reported to be related to a trial agent.

    In a systematic review and meta-analysis of 5 randomized clinical trials, treatment with the combination of a MEK and BRAF inhibitor was associated with an increased risk of pulmonary embolism, a decrease in left ventricular ejection fraction, and arterial hypertension compared with BRAF inhibitor monotherapy.

Reference(s):

- Courand PY, Berger M, Bouali A, Harbaoui B, Lantelme P, Dalle S. Cardiac Effects of BRAF and MEK Inhibitors: Mechanisms and Clinical Management. Curr Oncol Rep. 2022 Mar;24(3):265-271. doi: 10.1007/s11912-022-01205-3. Epub 2022 Feb 1. PMID: 35102484.
- Falchook GS, Lewis KD, Infante JR, Gordon MS, Vogelzang NJ, DeMarini DJ, Sun P, Moy C, Szabo SA, Roadcap LT, Peddareddigari VG, Lebowitz PF, Le NT, Burris HA 3rd, Messersmith WA, O'Dwyer PJ, Kim KB, Flaherty K, Bendell JC, Gonzalez R, Kurzrock R, Fecher LA. Activity of the oral MEK inhibitor trametinib in patients with advanced melanoma: a phase 1 dose-escalation trial. Lancet Oncol. 2012 Aug;13(8):782-9. doi: 10.1016/S1470-2045(12)70269-3. Epub 2012 Jul 16. PMID: 22805292; PMCID: PMC4109286.
- Mincu RI, Mahabadi AA, Michel L, Mrotzek SM, Schadendorf D, Rassaf T, Totzeck M. Cardiovascular Adverse Events Associated With BRAF and MEK Inhibitors: A Systematic Review and Meta-analysis. JAMA Netw Open. 2019 Aug 2;2(8):e198890. doi: 10.1001/jamanetworkopen.2019.8890. PMID: 31397860; PMCID: PMC6692687.
- Robert C, Grob JJ, Stroyakovskiy D, Karaszewska B, Hauschild A, Levchenko E, ChiarionSileni V, Schachter J, Garbe C, Bondarenko I, Gogas H, Mandalá M, Haanen JBAG, Lebbé C, Mackiewicz A, Rutkowski P, Nathan PD, Ribas A, Davies MA, Flaherty KT, Burgess P, Tan M, Gasal E, Voi M, Schadendorf D, Long GV. Five-Year Outcomes with Dabrafenib plus Trametinib in Metastatic Melanoma. N Engl J Med. 2019 Aug 15;381(7):626-636. doi: 10.1056/NEJMoa1904059. Epub 2019 Jun 4. PMID: 31166680.

95. Which of the following drugs used in the treatment of T315I-positive chronic myeloid leukemia is associated with arterial and venous thromboembolic events?

    A. Bevacizumab

    B. Osimertinib

    C. Ponatinib

    D. Ruxolitinib

    Ponatinib is an oral tyrosine kinase inhibitor indicated for the treatment of T315I-positive chronic myeloid leukemia (CML) (chronic phase, accelerated phase, or blast phase) or T3151-positive Philadelphia chromosome positive (Ph+) acute lymphoblastic leukemia, the treatment of patients with chronic phase CML with resistance or intolerance to at least two prior kinase inhibitors, and the treatment of patients with accelerated phase or blast phase CML or Ph+ ALL for whom no other kinase inhibitors are indicated. In a phase 2 trial of heavily pretreated patients who had CML or Ph+ ALL with resistance to or unacceptable side effects from dasatinib or nilotinib or who had the BCR-ABL T3151 mutation, ponatinib was found to be associated with a higher risk of arterial and venous thromboembolic events. Cardiovascular, cerebrovascular, and peripheral vascular events that were considered by the site investigator to be at least possibly related to ponatinib were observed in 2.2%, 0.7%, and 1.6% of patients, respectively. Other major adverse events associated with ponatinib include hypertension, pancreatitis, neuropathy, ocular toxicity, hemorrhage, fluid retention, cardiac arrhythmias, myelosuppression, tumor lysis syndrome, reversible posterior leukoencephalopathy syndrome, impaired wound healing, gastrointestinal perforation, and embryo-fetal toxicity.

Reference(s):

- Cortes JE, Kim DW, Pinilla-Ibarz J, le Coutre P, Paquette R, Chuah C, Nicolini FE, Apperley JF, Khoury HJ, Talpaz M, DiPersio J, DeAngelo DJ, Abruzzese E, Rea D, Baccarani M, Müller MC, Gambacorti-Passerini C, Wong S, Lustgarten S, Rivera VM, Clackson T, Turner CD, Haluska FG, Guilhot F, Deininger MW, Hochhaus A, Hughes T, Goldman JM, Shah NP, Kantarjian H; PACE Investigators. A phase 2 trial of ponatinib in Philadelphia chromosome-positive leukemias. N Engl J Med. 2013 Nov 7;369(19):1783-96. doi: 10.1056/NEJMoa1306494. Epub 2013 Nov 1. PMID: 24180494; PMCID: PMC3886799.
- Cortes JE, Kim DW, Pinilla-Ibarz J, le Coutre PD, Paquette R, Chuah C, Nicolini FE, Apperley JF, Khoury HJ, Talpaz M, DeAngelo DJ, Abruzzese E, Rea D, Baccarani M, Müller MC, Gambacorti-Passerini C, Lustgarten S, Rivera VM, Haluska FG, Guilhot F, Deininger MW, Hochhaus A, Hughes TP, Shah NP, Kantarjian HM. Ponatinib efficacy and safety in Philadelphia chromosome-positive leukemia: final 5-year results of the phase 2 PACE trial. Blood. 2018 Jul 26;132(4):393-404. doi: 10.1182/blood-2016-09-739086. Epub 2018 Mar 22. PMID: 29567798; PMCID: PMC6071555.

96. Which of the following drugs used in the treatment of metastatic, epidermal growth factor receptor (EGFR) T790M mutation-positive, non-small cell lung cancer is associated with QT interval prolongation and cardiomyopathy?

    A. Afatinib

    B. Dacomitinib

    C. Erlotinib

    D. Osimertinib

    Osimertinib has been associated with a number of adverse cardiac events. In an interrogation of the U.S. Food and Drug Administration Adverse Events Reporting System (FAERS) pharmacovigilance database it was found that the reporting odds ratio (ROR) (95% confidence interval) for cardiac failure, atrial fibrillation (AF), QT prolongation, myocardial infarction, and pericardial effusion due to osimertinib versus all other drugs in FAERS was 5.4 (4.2 to 7.1), 4.0 (2.8 to 5.8), 11.2 (7.9 to 15.8), 1.6 (0.9 to 2.6), and 8.2 (4.8 to 14), respectively. The ROR (95% CI) for cardiac failure, AF, QT prolongation, myocardial infarction, and pericardial effusion in comparing osimertinib versus other epidermal growth factor receptor (EGFR)-tyrosine kinase inhibitors was 2.2 (1.5 to 3.2), 2.1 (1.3 to 3.5), 6.6 (3.4 to 12.8), 1.2 (0.6 to 2.3), and 1.6 (0.8 to 3.3).

    Afatinib is indicated for the treatment of patients with metastatic non-small cell lung cancer (NSCLC) whose tumors have non-resistant EGFR mutations. Dacomitinib is another kinase inhibitor indicated for the treatment of patients with metastatic NSCLC with EGFR exon 19 deletion or exon 21 L858R substitution mutations. Erlotinib is approved for maintenance treatment of patients with locally advanced or metastatic NSCLC whose disease has not progressed after four cycles of platinum-based chemotherapy; treatment of locally advanced or metastatic NSCLC after failure of at least one prior chemotherapy regimen; and treatment of patients with locally advanced, unresectable, or metastatic pancreatic cancer in combination with gemcitabine.

Reference(s):

- Anand K, Ensor J, Trachtenberg B, Bernicker EH. Osimertinib-Induced Cardiotoxicity: A Retrospective Review of the FDA Adverse Events Reporting System (FAERS). JACC CardioOncol. 2019 Dec 17;1(2):172-178. doi: 10.1016/j.jaccao.2019.10.006. PMID: 34396179; PMCID: PMC8352117.

97. Which of the following types of cancer is associated with non-bacterial thrombotic endocarditis?

    A. Glioblastoma multiforme

    B. Lymphoma

    C. Melanoma

    D. Pancreas

    Nonbacterial thrombotic endocarditis (NBTE), also known as marantic endocarditis, is a phenomenon due to hypercoagulability that typically affects patients with underlying adenocarcinoma, often of pancreatic origin. It is commonly confused with infective endocarditis, which is due to an infectious etiology. Patients can be asymptomatic, whereas others can present with a thromboembolic event (ie, ischemic stroke), cardiac valve dysfunction, murmurs, or heart failure symptoms.

Reference(s):

- Piovanelli B, Rovetta R, Bonadei I, Vizzardi E, D'Aloia A, Metra M. Nonbacterial thrombotic endocarditis in pancreatic cancer. Monaldi Arch Chest Dis. 2013 Dec;80(4):189-92. doi: 10.4081/monaldi.2013.5236. PMID: 25087296.
- Spurgeon L, Ispoglou S. Non-bacterial thrombotic endocarditis in pancreatic cancer and other high-risk malignancies: the case for prophylactic treatment. Oxf Med Case Reports. 2021 Nov 25;2021(11):omab110. doi: 10.1093/omcr/omab110. PMID: 34858625; PMCID: PMC8633644.

98. A 65-year-old male with Philadelphia chromosome-positive acute lymphoblastic leukemia on treatment presents with worsening dyspnea on exertion. A chest X-ray shows a new right-sided pleural effusion and an enlarged cardiac silhouette. Which of the following cancer therapeutics would explain his clinical presentation?

    A. Dasatinib

    B. Imatinib

    C. Nilotinib

    D. Ponatinib

Dasatinib is considered an effective drug in imatinib-resistant chronic myeloid leukemia. Although reported to be well-tolerated, severe events such as pleural or pericardial effusion have been reported at a variety of doses. This has been replicated worldwide with Japanese studies showing more frequent cardiac side effects in patients with CML and GIST treated with dasatinib compared to imatinib.

Reference(s):

- Krauth MT, Herndlhofer S, Schmook MT, Mitterbauer-Hohendanner G, Schlögl E, Valent P. Extensive pleural and pericardial effusion in chronic myeloid leukemia during treatment with dasatinib at 100 mg or 50 mg daily. Haematologica. 2011 Jan;96(1):163-6. doi: 10.3324/haematol.2010.030494. Epub 2010 Oct 7. PMID: 20934998; PMCID: PMC3012781.
- Motokawa T, Ikeda S, Ueno Y, Eguchi M, Minami T, Kawano H, Kobayashi K, Imaizumi Y, Maemura K. Comparison of Dasatinib- and Imatinib-Related Cardiotoxic Adverse Events in Japanese Patients With Chronic Myeloid Leukemia and Gastrointestinal Stromal Tumor. Circ Rep. 2021 Nov 16;4(1):1-8. doi: 10.1253/circrep.CR-21-0140. PMID: 35083382; PMCID: PMC8710638.

99. Which of the following drugs is an FLT-3 inhibitor associated with QT interval prolongation approved for the treatment of adult patients who have relapsed or refractory acute myeloid leukemia (AML)?

A. Cabozantinib

B. Dabrafenib

C. Gilteritinib

D. Sorafenib

In a phase 3 trial involving patients with relapsed or refractory AML with mutations in the FMS-like tyrosine kinase 3 gene (FLT3), gilteritinib was shown to significantly improve survival and achieve higher percentages of patients with remission compared with salvage chemotherapy. QT interval prolongation attributed to gilteritinib occurred in 12 patients (4.9%), but only 1 patient (0.4%) had a maximum post-baseline increase in the mean QT interval (corrected using Fridericia's formula) of more than 500 milliseconds.

Reference(s):

- Perl AE, Martinelli G, Cortes JE, Neubauer A, Berman E, Paolini S, Montesinos P, Baer MR, Larson RA, Ustun C, Fabbiano F, Erba HP, Di Stasi A, Stuart R, Olin R, Kasner M, Ciceri F, Chou WC, Podoltsev N, Recher C, Yokoyama H, Hosono N, Yoon SS, Lee JH, Pardee T, Fathi AT, Liu C, Hasabou N, Liu X, Bahceci E, Levis MJ. Gilteritinib or Chemotherapy for Relapsed or Refractory FLT3-Mutated AML. N Engl J Med. 2019 Oct 31;381(18):1728-1740. doi: 10.1056/NEJMoa1902688. Erratum in: N Engl J Med. 2022 May 12;386(19):1868. PMID: 31665578.

100. A 67-year-old male with history of hypertension and asymptomatic paroxysmal atrial fibrillation is diagnosed with mantle cell lymphoma. In addition to easy bruising, he also has intermittent nausea resulting from his malignancy. His oncologist recommends starting ibrutinib. Within two weeks of starting ibrutinib, the patient develops symptomatic atrial fibrillation with rapid ventricular response. Considering potential drug-drug interaction, which of the following medications would be most appropriate to manage his atrial fibrillation?

A. Amiodarone

B. Diltiazem

C. Dronedarone

D. Metoprolol

Due to interactions with cytochrome P450 CYP3A4 system, the concomitant use of non-dihydropyridine calcium channel blockers, amiodarone, and dronedarone can lead to elevated levels of ibrutinib and subsequent toxicity. There are no significant interactions with beta blockers.

Reference(s):

- Essa H, Lodhi T, Dobson R, Wright D, Lip GYH. How to Manage Atrial Fibrillation Secondary to Ibrutinib. JACC CardioOncol. 2021 Mar 16;3(1):140-144. doi: 10.1016/j.jaccao.2020.11.016. PMID: 34396314; PMCID: PMC8352308.
- Ganatra S, Sharma A, Shah S, Chaudhry GM, Martin DT, Neilan TG, Mahmood SS, Barac A, Groarke JD, Hayek SS, Dani S, Venesy D, Patten R, Nohria A. Ibrutinib-Associated Atrial Fibrillation. JACC Clin Electrophysiol. 2018 Dec;4(12):1491-1500. doi: 10.1016/j.jacep.2018.06.004. Epub 2018 Aug 29. PMID: 30573111.

www.ingramcontent.com/pod-product-compliance
Ingram Content Group UK Ltd.
Pitfield, Milton Keynes, MK11 3LW, UK
UKHW020655041026
15590UKWH00001B/284

9 781735 644226